Dear

How to Get Laid Using Your Intuition

May all your Dominant Dreams

Susanna Brisk

Come true ♡

Edited by Sunny Megatron

XO

Intuitively,

Susanna Brisk

This material is the intellectual property of Susanna Brisk, Sexual Intuitive® and cannot be shared or reproduced without express permission from the author.

For media, as well as coaching enquiries, please email sexualintuitive@gmail.com.

ISBN-13: 978-0692070185

For M.M.—Thank you for being living proof of what I believed in my bones.

"I believe in intuitions and inspirations...I sometimes *feel* that I am right. I do not *know* that I am."
Albert Einstein

"My intuition is telling me they'll be better days."
J. Cole

Contents

Consent Forward

This book is not intended to tell you what to do, but as a tool to straighten out self-limiting beliefs, and confirm what you didn't know you knew. Once you gain the 'inner knowing' that directs you towards people who are interested in exploring sexually with you, consent is an explicit way to confirm your intuition. Without their consent, your intuition is not validated. Overriding someone's resistance to sleeping with you is not the same as being Dominant.

Any time you have to override anyone, it's not consent, and therefore, besides being morally questionable, is not a sustainable approach to getting laid. There's no joy to be gained in getting something that is not freely and enthusiastically given. Being forthright and specific about what is going to occur, including giving someone the opportunity to say no at any time, does not 'ruin the moment.' In fact, it makes each moment that much hotter when someone is given the space to choose to say, "Fuck *yes.*"

Prologue: You Already Got This

I didn't have the worst childhood, but I can say with certainty that life pretty much sucked until I started getting laid. Sure, there were some fun times growing up as a Russian Jew in Australia; koalas, latkes, some rousing piano recitals... but once I got older and that cock went in, it hit some kind of magic button that said, "Everything will now and forever be okay." Who knew happiness was lurking up behind my cervix?

For a while there, I thought my love of sex and all things kinky was a sign I was a 'sex addict.' (It wasn't.) It turns out that *wanting* to get laid is a good thing, but you wouldn't know it if you're looking for clues in our culture. We're inundated with contradictory tips, tricks, and techniques that may 'drive your lover crazy' *literally.* We've been taught to hold it like a basket, suck the tip like it's ice cream, and lick the shape of the alphabet, but how are we supposed to know in what font?

You don't have to have a high sex drive or a low one to be 'normal.' You can just be you, wadded up tissues and all. Despite what you might have been taught by your parents, your church, or your friends, being horny is your greatest ally. If your desire is inconsistent, that's understandable considering your parents, your church, and your friends. For now, it's okay just to *want* to want sex, despite the seeming evidence that Lucy/Lucifer will snatch the football away at the last moment.

In this book I'll show you that most of what you believe about getting laid is not helping you. This is *especially* true when it comes to some kind of magical pickup tips/tricks/techniques that work to melt anyone's panties/jockstrap/loincloth. The majority of what we've been taught about sex is a lie and what we believe about ourselves a distortion—believe it or not, *this is the good news*. Getting laid is supposed to be natural and easy, and it will be, once you parse out and brush away all that has made it seem difficult.

The reason you haven't figured out how to get laid with the regularity you want is **not** a failure on your part. It's **not** a lack of intelligence, charm, or looks that has brought you to this juncture. In fact, it may have been frustrating for you to watch people with far less attributes than you sail towards the fuck-appointments of their dreams. *What do they know that you don't?*

At this point dating may be fraught with so much frustration and misery (with a side of hot rage) that you've given up. By the end of this book, I promise you'll have the tools to get *most of your sexual needs met, most of the time*. I know this because I've been where you are, and because of my own journey, have helped thousands of others find their true sexual expression, both through my writing and Sexual Intuitive® coaching.

America is based on the idea that if you search far and wide, and throw down enough cold cash, we got a cure for what ails ya. They've told us to text/not text, be logical/follow your heart, wait/fuck—in order to sell us the cure. Except that in order for us to buy what they're peddling, *they* have to convince us there's something 'off' about us that needs fixing. We're all drooling morons and only their product/service/idea can save us.

It's the same implication used in advertising that your looks, life, and experiences are somehow inferior to what *is out there somewhere*. Most of the advice dispensed about sex, love, and relationships comes with the idea that you need help because **you don't know what the fuck you're doing.**

I'm here to tell you that you *do*… just not in the way you think. Together we will hack into the inner guidance system that will show you the next right action, based on both the situation, and the person, you find yourself in. You need never second-guess yourself again. (To help you navigate, you'll find a glossary of terms, acronyms, and context of words the way I use them at the end of this book.)

But before you can begin to access your Sexual Intuition, you have to get real. Essentially, you have to be willing to look inside yourself before you can look inside someone else.

My favorite analogy for clients is let's say you have a physical storage space full of junk you haven't gone into for years and are now committed to clearing out. When you first walk in and switch on the light it's a shitshow; more disorganized than you remembered, with moldy boxes full of horrifying childhood knick-knacks you're somehow still attached to.

Was there any less mess a moment ago, when it was locked up in the dark behind a heavy door? Of course not, it just seemed *more manageable* because you couldn't see it.

Investigating that room means taking inventory of how you've been operating in the areas of sex and dating to figure out and discard, not what *defines* you, only what no longer serves. You don't have to part with that blacklight Bruce Lee poster, I promise. So let's begin by bravely flipping on the lights...

Part 1.0: Getting Real

1.1: To Get Laid Stop Focusing on Getting Laid

Let's start by recalibrating what we think of as 'getting laid' (it'll help you get laid, I promise). If you're predominantly hetero, you may take for granted that sex happens when a penis enters a vagina and hey presto, fucking. But fucking equals different things to different fuckers. If we feel we've been 'bait and switched' in dating and relationships it might be time to switch [what we think of] as the bait. That starts with not treating penetrative boning as some kind of finish line we're desperate to cross.

If you identify as any version of LGBTQI, you already know that getting laid is a much broader experience than penetration. Women who have sex with women know fingers, mouths, friction, kissing, and toys can bring a dizzying array of cumly delights. Likewise, gay men understand that hand, mouth, and/or any combo of ass-play totally 'count.' Gender fluid people have found endlessly creative ways to get off. It's mostly the straights that have this whole attachment to a penetrative endgame and it's not helping, despite what you may have been taught by Setting-Goals-Is-The-Key-To-Success-Bro.

Kissing, mutual handies, cunni- or any other lingus, are all sex. Believe it or not, even gazing into someone's eyes that you're attracted to can release the same yummy fuck chemicals into the brain, like serotonin, dopamine, norepinephrine, and oxytocin. Not everyone wants to go to pound town every single time they're attracted to someone, which should start to help you understand that it has *nothing to do with you* when they don't, or in the past when they didn't. You'll see that you can attract folks who want the same things you want.

Even those sexperiences you considered clumsy and unsatisfying follow a forward trajectory because each is a progression towards the *kind* of sex you want in the future. In the world of sex, dating, love, and relationships there's no such thing as a mistake, there's only progress. The way you know that something was supposed to happen *is that it did*. Once you tune in more accurately to your intuition, you will understand what there was to learn, and move on.

If you feel disappointed by the duration, frequency, and/or sanity of your past encounters, welcome to adulthood! One way to change the frustration about past liaisons is to reframe them. You wouldn't build a castle on a sinkhole, so it's important that your next forays into the dating world are not built on what you consider to be 'failures.' Start to believe that every single time you had a crush on someone, dared to flirt, or even got your heart broken after a frantic finger blast, it was a win. Everything counts, nothing matters, and once more into the breach, brave one, let's go!

A recent survey by Forbes magazine claims that while most (predominantly hetero, racially unidentified) cis men and women still prefer penetrative vaginal sex to any other sex acts, there's also a high degree of interest in non-penetrative acts of intimacy such as 'watching a partner undress,' 'creating a romantic room,' and 'cuddling.' While this book was not written just to help you get more cuddles, you will figure out how to get laid in a way that feels satisfying and complete.

According to a recent study by the University of Indiana, "While vaginal intercourse is still the most common sexual behavior reported by adults, many sexual events do not involve intercourse and include only partnered masturbation or oral sex." In other words, lots of things feel just as good as 'traditional' fucking—insert Tab A into Slot B—getting to 'third base' is not a failure on your part.

Your first assignment is to stop seeing potential partners as gatekeepers to their genitals, or hurdles in the way of hurtling over the finish line ribbon to collect your penetration trophy. In this way you'll make space for a new, more effective approach that you will design shortly.

There's no doubt we've been lied to when it comes to sex and dating. There is a misconception that if you didn't either 'close the deal' and/or 'live happily ever after' then it was a waste of your time. Sexy events you believe 'didn't count' or even fantasies you've had contain useful information to build on. Now that you know there's more than one way to get laid, we can talk about how your instincts will guide you to every nasty one of them.

DIY: *Your first assignment is to write about* **what worked** *about your past encounters with people, even if you have gotten used to seeing some of these encounters or relationships as 'failures.' Rather than using your past experiences to back up a negative preconception about what sex/love/dating is like, focus on what was good and fun, so you can build on those qualities in the future. You may want to use the template, "When I was with _____, one of my favorite things was _____, and in future I want more of _____.*

1.2: **What Do You Fuck With?**

As of this writing, there's no college curriculum called *How to Bang Good 101*. Most of us stumble into a strategy, which then becomes 'that thing I do.' When a fuck strategy doesn't evolve over time, it's because we have no consciousness around it. If we don't understand where we've been coming from, we can't effectively choose something that might work better. We settle for a 'throw the spaghetti at the wall and see what sticks' approach to dating, instead of something more intentional.

What I've noticed through having thousands of people confide in me over multiple decades, is that most will settle on *one* of three ways to choose willing sex participants—guided by the *Cerebral*, the *Emotional*, or the *Genital.* People land on predominantly *one* of these, at the expense of the others. Unfortunately, this also limits the power of the intuitive sense to take over, in ways I will explain later. For now, just be aware that for intuition to be activated, you can factor in the *Cerebral*, the *Emotional* and the *Genital*, so you can supersede them in ways that may not make immediate sense.

The *Cerebral* approach is when we date or fuck someone because we think we're supposed to go for someone *like* them. They're a practical or convenient choice, have qualities we've decided are admirable, or we believe they're 'hot enough' to fulfill some projected criteria. We can mentally see ourselves with a two-dimensional *idea* of them, which gives us a positive *idea* about ourselves.

Often when clients come to me for coaching it's because they're aware of something about their sexual desires that feels really fucking urgent, either in the kind of people they choose to be with/pursue or a dissatisfaction with the person they're with. Sometimes this somewhat painful situation has come about because at some moment they chose to override their instincts with intellect.

Consider *Cerebral* Dave, a highly successful mid-30's professional in the IT field who hired me to coach him because his encounters with women had been confusing and awkward. Despite being an appealing man with a laconic sense of humor, he despaired of ever finding a willing fuck-partner again. Even if he did, past experiences made Dave afraid that his body would betray him, as it had before.

As we worked together, it became apparent that Dave had never made an irrational decision in his life. Where he lived, what he drove, and his career were a series of strategic steps all leading up to a meticulously planned-for retirement. I didn't ask Dave his credit score, but I sensed it was impressive.

Dave thought of women as irrational, untrustworthy and hard to understand (ha).

When I asked him whether he'd had sex, he wasn't sure if having sex with a paid companion 'counted.' He complained of being 'in his head' even in the midst of acts that made him horny when he thought or masturbated about them. The realness of an actual woman was off-putting when compared to his (porn-fueled) fantasies. Dave needed to get his head around this one area he couldn't 'get his head around.'

Beyond any kind of reasonableness, we came up with a plan for Dave to visit another country, where women were more forthright and even downright aggressive—an energy that turned Dave on. This rather irrational decision was made *beyond* what we intellectually researched about women in that country, who they were and the ethnicity of men they preferred, but rather from the 'gut.' Dave went on his trip and did indeed get laid with one of these ladies (she is planning to come out and see him, last I heard). He was also able to return to his hometown USA with newfound confidence that he could replicate those results in another dialect.

Emotional Stella was waiting for 'the right guy' who would be a 'gentleman' and 'treat her right.' Yet she went for guys much younger than herself, millennials who were not interested in the more old-school kind of wooing she craved, leading to a state of almost continual heartbreak. She believed in a rigid structure of dates to try to suss out a dude's character before she slept with him (1. Coffee 2. Dinner 3. Fingerbang.) She trusted only how she *felt* for guidance, desperate for indications that someone was going to cherish her, ignoring the (sometimes) obvious signs that the dudes she chose weren't able to cherish anyone.

By the age of 50, never married, and without any 'successful' relationships under her belt, Stella had been disappointed so many times that in response her dating rules got even more stringent. Her strategy of 'holding out' for a 'soulmate' would waver when she got horny enough. At those times, she would drop all her boundaries, throw herself at an inappropriate *Genital*, and starting the cycle of heartbreak yet again.

Emotionals pursue based on what their 'heart' is telling them, even though the heart is actually a collection of muscles that Westerners imbue with feels. (According to Indonesians, the seat of feelings is the liver, leading to the poetic "I love you with all my liver.") A heart (or liver)-centered approach is great, except when it's empowered as the sole decision maker for whom you pick, and what you get up to with them. Just because you love someone, doesn't mean you're going to love fucking them.

Emotionals are not all women, and don't necessarily present as emo in the rest of their lives. They may be as detached as sharks when it comes to business or friendships, they just use sentiment-driven criteria for sexual attraction. The challenge with being an *Emotional* is that sentimentalizing sex leaves out the dirty, messy portions that make it so much fun! It's also difficult for *Emotionals* to make peace with having sex without being in love, putting undue pressure on a partner that makes their liver quiver.

For Stella, it meant trusting her instincts instead of ignoring them and getting carried away on a sea of emotion. Stella had to let go of the fantasy of what a relationship could be versus hearing what this real life human being was clearly communicating (by using tools I will give you later in this book.) There was always a point even very early on, where Stella *knew* how things were going to play out. By paying attention to this *knowing*, she was able to make better choices for herself, be direct in her communication, and have more consistent, fulfilling sex with guys she was still attracted to that factored in whether or not they were DTR (Down To Relationship).

Genitals are those driven by hormones, pheromones, and what's below the belt as opposed to between the ears or in the heart space. *Genitals* rely on visual cues, rarely being able to sense folks beyond the superficial. While *Genitals* may get laid often because of sheer commitment, the trap is that sex can become mechanical or rote, and sooner or later, as age or other factors catch up with them, their concept of sexuality stays immature or limited. *Genitals* may use silicone slabs with holes or vibrating sex toys when a human is not available, and this may feel like an inferior substitute. (There is nothing wrong with Fleshlights, sex dolls, and VR sex, but this book is intended to get you laid IRL.)

Veronica The *Genital* was a mental health professional, yet she made questionable decisions when it came to sex. She slept with addicts who barely expressed an interest in her, and celebrities she felt were 'better' than she was. She finally got fired from her job in a treatment center for having sex with a female client. Her trysts ended not just in heartbreak, but legal action. (Someone needs to give Veronica her own TV show.)

Veronica was driven completely by *Genital* attraction, unable to bring in her otherwise strong intellect or kind heart to find someone *appropro*. She identified as a 'sex addict' and couldn't visualize integrating her high sex drive with any kind of manageable existence. She pathologized her enjoyment of sex, without accepting that any of her needs might be valid, and even viable! Veronica needed to learn a less polarized, black-and-white view of what was possible for her. In order to be a functional human being, she had to integrate all her needs and desires by painstakingly uncovering what they were, then allowing herself to believe she could meet them.

If your Head, Heart, and *Geni*s are consistently not aligned, you're probably using *one* sensory system at a time and missing out on the benefits of the rest. Any one of these might get you laid, but in order to ward off either shitty sex or no sex at all, you'll need to go deeper. In this book, I will show you how to strengthen your *Cerebral-Emotional-Genital* with something even more powerful, perceptive, and juicy—your GUT.

To have earth-shattering, planet-realigning, galaxy-exploding sex, you need a strong Brain-Heart-Dick connection. Or obviously, as it applies, a Brain-Heart-Pussy connection. You can have a Brain-Heart-Whatever-Combo-You-Got connection; what's most important is that you function in an ideal state of flow within yourself. Take a moment now to consider what motivated your choices in the past, and how that tunnel vision might have limited you.

I once had a client come to me complaining of ED. Rufus had been with Julia for three months, had never encountered the issue before, and was freaked out that he was in his twenties and his equipment was failing him. I listened to him talk listlessly about his girlfriend for a good half-hour before offering him my intuitive hit.

"Can I be honest?" I prefaced, even though I tend to attract the kind of client that prefers honesty.

"Of course," he replied.

"It sounds like you don't want to fuck her anymore."

He beamed. "I *don't* want to fuck her anymore."

Once we came to this truth that resonated for him, we could begin to uncover and investigate what kind of *needs* Rufus had and how he could get them met, from a place of freedom, instead of obligation. Sometimes a low libido or something else you diagnose as dysfunction is not a sign something is horribly wrong, but rather that you have a good *Cerebral/ Emotional/Genital* connection. Let's build on that!

A word on (small g) genitals- whether you have a cock or a vulva; or if you're queer, trans, or another gender beyond the binary, you are welcome here. What you have in your pants and how you prefer to fuck are unrelated, what matters is how you align your approach with your needs (more about this soon.) You can identify as a boy with a pussy, or a chick with a dick, or some other politically iffy lexicon—activists like Buck Angel (the original 'man with a pussy') and Bailey Jay ('rebel without a cunt') will tell you it's not for anyone to police what you call yourself. When I use the terms male/female, boy/girl, man/woman, I'm referring to the energy of 'masculine' and 'feminine,' which are increasingly understood as fluid concepts, and appear in endless configurations. Likewise, if you're a cis-gender man or woman who just wants to get some pussy, I won't hold it against you.

1.3: There's No Such Thing As A Negative Sexual Urge

At the beginning of one of my workshops I gave participants different essential oils to smell and asked them to pick a favorite. They had no trouble with it. They didn't balk, get defensive or apologize for their lascivious love for lavender, their perverted preference for peppermint, not to mention that *dirty* eucalyptus obsession that almost cost them a happy marriage. Yet, when it comes to our own sexual tastes, some of us have a hard time even identifying and accepting what turns us on most.

We don't have to argue with ourselves about our desires, because they don't say anything more about us than happening to like a lemon scent. It doesn't really *mean* anything if we favor 'eucalyptus' over 'sage.' Substitute 'anal sex' for 'eucalyptus' and 'nipple clamps' for 'sage' and suddenly we get all *judgy*.

"Uh, I'm more of a *clary sage* person myself. I just can't get with these *sage* freaks, brah."

Women especially can have wildly different preferences at different times—for both sex and sage—depending on hormonal changes. In this book, you will learn to let your instincts guide you towards picking the right time to initiate eucalyptus, partly by noticing when someone has olfactory overload.

I also use the ice cream analogy with clients. When I ask someone what their favorite ice cream is, they rarely ruminate.

"You like mint chip better than vanilla?"

"Yeah."

"And what does that say about you?"

"Nothing, I guess. Just that I like mint chip."

"Exactly. So, start thinking about your sexual tastes that way, without assigning any *meaning* to them. You're just a mint chip kinda guy, Muriel..."

In my experience, when clients or friends struggle with recurring thoughts or fantasies about something they see as 'taboo,' they're afraid to 'give in' to them lest they become some fuck maniac prowling dairy aisles waiting to stick their fingers in unsuspecting tubs of Rocky Road. (They probably won't.)

Your fantasies are fuel to give you more information about yourself, so pay attention. You can learn to think of any 'odd' or 'fucked up' fantasies you have as a kind of superhighway to fulfilling a basic need specific only to you (you will learn to identify these needs in a later chapter). The point is not the dental fetish you've been secretly nursing, but the fact that for whatever reason, watching someone brush, floss, or lick their teeth fulfills a certain core craving for you. It scratches an itch nothing else can reach, is satisfying in a way nothing else can be, and there is absolutely nothing wrong with that!

Just because you fantasize about something, doesn't mean you necessarily have any desire or intention to engage in it in real life, so why would you deprive yourself of a fantasy? And if at a later point you find a willing partner, what's wrong with a little consensual flossing between adults?

While it makes no sense to deny yourself full and complete mental expression, *not every sexual urge should be acted on.* Can a child consent? No. Can an animal consent? No. Can someone incapacitated by drugs, alcohol, a diminished mental state consent, or the possibility of being fired/promoted consent? No.

If your fantasies include some form of non-consent, fighting against them will only warp them into something much, much worse. There are ways to find expression to these intense cravings that are positive and healthy, even if that doesn't make you Johnny Wholesome. As long as you're living in reality, *nothing is wrong with imagination*, no matter what it is. You can even find partners willing to consensually roleplay some of these scenarios with you! If you believe your filthy thoughts make you despicable to Jesus, Jehovah, or Joseph Smith, then you have some work to do to define a loving higher power that created you with your own quirks for a reason.

When you attach a stigma to your fantasies they can fester into a darker pattern of compulsion, or what is referred to by the term 'sex addiction.' Intuitively speaking, sex addiction is an absence of the light of awareness being shone on a person's inner life. Dr. Chris Donaghue, the sex therapist, broadcaster, and author of *Sex Between The Lines*, believes that 'sex addiction' is not a valid diagnosis and I agree. In my experience as both a human and a coach, I believe that lumping the idea of being 'addicted to sex' with other process addictions—behaviors like gambling, rather than substances like alcohol—is a mistake. While patterns of porn use, masturbation, and casual sex can get compulsive, they can also be steadied if desires are normalized, investigated, and accepted, instead of being demonized and pushed into the shadows.

Many great artists have explored the darker sides of sexuality without disappearing into permanent ruin. "The Story of O" is an S&M classic, published under the pseudonym Pauline Réage in 1954, known as the original 50 Shades of Grey. I know it as the book I masturbated to so much in the late 1980's that the cover came off. (Back before the internet, we whacked analog.)

In "The Story of the Eye," Georges Bataille's literary masterpiece, a couple copulate next to the dead body of a priest, with the woman eventually inserting his enucleated eye into her vagina, and that's only after all the other necrophilia, bestiality, and eroticized suicide.

Good times!

Life can imitate art without mirroring it exactly, just as porn is porn, and not life. If dark sexual fantasies are part of your 'art' why not indulge in them? Not everyone has to go full Marquis de Sade and act that shit out.

No one can arrest you for the contents of your head, and even if they do, a recent legal precedent says they have to release you eventually. New York's 'Cannibal Cop' was the sensational case of a police officer who hung out in flesh-eating fetish communities online, until he was arrested and jailed in 2013 for sounding like he might do something about it with his real-life partner. His conviction was overturned in 2015, because regardless of his overall character, the guy *never actually did anything*.

We all have the right to fantasize about *whatever* we want to—the point of using your imagination is no one gets hurt. [1] Make your brain the ultimate democracy, allow yourself true freedom of thought, without censorship, and you will develop the confident glow of being okay with what you think about.

Accepting your sexual tastes as normal and natural is the first cornerstone of operating intuitively, both inside and on the way to the bedroom. What you're into and believe you're *not* into will change and expand over time, just as when you were a kid you may have liked bubblegum ice cream, and now your tastes have matured to salted caramel. You wouldn't try to mold your frozen treat preferences into what you *should* enjoy. A liberating way to think of it is, "For today, I like what I like, but tomorrow I may want something different." Except pistachio. No one likes pistachio, you weirdo.

[1] If you find yourself seeking out images or films of real children or people being non-consensually tortured, please seek professional help with someone who doesn't have to shame you, but can support you in identifying a way to express your sexuality that doesn't damage real life humans.

1.4: Torture Loops and Psychic Shrapnel

Trusting your intuition is different than thinking something must be true because you *really* believe it. During the course of a day (let alone a lifetime) we accumulate thousands of stories we could compellingly believe. We receive data and we organize it, because who doesn't love a pattern? A is *true*, and A is *always* followed by B and *therefore* C, and around and around it goes. I call these Torture Loops.

In terms of how we perceive ourselves, most of us reside in the area between Unworthy (someone who does not see their own value) and Delusional (someone who has an inflated view of themselves) called Human. Some of what we have in common with other humans of assorted shapes, sizes, races, genders, and income brackets are our unfortunate habit of getting stuck in Torture Loops. Unlike a raccoon that can get its paw stuck in a literal metal trap, we are the only species smart enough to do this to ourselves mentally. Yay!

Torture Loops are obsessive, relentless, and can include some combination of:

◆ Replaying conversations with people.

41

- Engaging in new mental conversations with people who are no longer in front of you or even *alive*.
- Resentment about things that happened anywhere between one minute and ninety years ago.
- Bitterness about someone else's success or (perceived) superiority.
- Shame about your own inferiority.
- Fear about something that hasn't happened yet, might never happen, and even if it did, you could probably deal with it.
- Judging other people's behavior without compassion.
- Too much compassion for others, and none for yourself.
- "He always…"
- "She never…"

A lot of our greatest convictions are formed when we're two-years-old, or eight, or fifteen, when someone larger than us tells us something about ourselves that actually has more to do with *them*, and in the absence of better information, we believe them. Sometimes, they're pre-verbal, like if mom had Post-Partum Depression and looked at you with ambivalence, and then you ran with it. Maybe mom just had gas that day, but we'll never know...

It's important to understand that Torture Loops feel comfortable at first, and were likely coping skills we developed to survive difficult situations. There is a comfort to being able to tie up our own behavior, our circumstances, and other people in a neat little bow. It's important to pay attention to when these coping mechanisms are no longer useful, so we can move beyond their limited worldview and into a more complicated and rich reality.

Torture Loops make life more manageable, until they make it less so. If you're reading this book, you're not a child anymore, and it's time to put a loving internalized adult in charge who can tell you you're safe enough to let these old paradigms go, a process outlined in the self-help classic *I'm Okay, You're Okay* by Thomas A. Harris. What Dr. Harris doesn't mention, is how this will help your internalized adult move towards the next rollicking orgasm.

You may have some pretty convincing Torture Loops going around sex. Consider these possible occurrences:

- I wasn't hard.

- I wasn't wet.
- He/she didn't want to go on a date.
- My cock is too small.
- My pussy is too big.
- My labia are too long.
- I came too fast.
- I couldn't come.
- That was bad sex.
- I didn't get to have sex.

In each of these cases it is not the actual facts that need be disturbing (embarrassing or unwanted in the moment, maybe), it's what we *decide* about it. It's when we add the *"And therefore..."* that we get into trouble.

In the case of the first two points (hardness and wetness respectively) there's a phenomenon studied and proven by Emily Nagoski PhD in her book *Come As You Are* called arousal non-concordance. Arousal non-concordance is basically your mind wanting one thing and your body not complying with the physiological response you thought was correct for that moment. Rather than adding the, *"And therefore..."* with some version of "THERE'S SOMETHING WRONG WITH ME," you could just accept it at face value. Okay, you weren't wet. NBD! Get some lube from the nightstand and move forward!

As someone who has had to contend with more than her fair share of Torture Loops, I'm very familiar. There's even a not so adorable cousin of the Torture Loop that I call Psychic Shrapnel. Shrapnel can be defined as the shot, fragments, or debris thrown out by an exploding shell, bomb, or landmine. The fragments that scatter when a bomb explodes are not part of the weapon, yet they can kill you.

Some of my clients come to me with sexual thoughts they find dark and highly disturbing. Sometimes these unwanted thoughts are violent. These are otherwise well-functioning people whose brains are snagging on a certain ugly idea like a hangnail. They wonder about their own character, or even their sanity, because what kind of person could compulsively return to awful thoughts over and over, and even masturbate over them?

The analogy that I use with clients is how in many towns you can stumble upon old train tracks that are no longer in use. They're only a few feet long and they don't lead anywhere, but the city or town has decided removing them carries too much hassle or expense. Psychic Shrapnel or really old Torture Loops are just like these unused tracks. You can learn to be less fascinated with them when you come across them accidentally. You don't have to deny their existence, but you can choose to see they don't lead anywhere, and go around them (more about this in the Fuck Trauma chapter.)

Unlike many therapists, I'm not concerned with analyzing every random, bizarre thought we have as human beings, especially when it comes to sex. We're all kinky as hell, so what?

It's important to develop a *neutral* relationship with your own dark side like, "Oh, there's that thought again…" Observe whether it has anything to teach you about your sexual preferences, and eventually it will either integrate into your life or go away entirely because there's no one to obsess about it anymore. Any hypnotherapist will tell you that the subconscious mind gets bored over time when we stop attaching an energetic charge to our thoughts, and moves on to more important things like #pugsofinstagram.

Have you ever sat across from people, on dates and otherwise, and watched them cycle through their Torture Loops, while also trying to circumnavigate landmines of Psychic Shrapnel? Most folks are on their best behavior, working to present a favorable image, and they would be perfectly happy if it weren't for 'what my ex-husband pulled' or 'when my ex-girlfriend cheated on me.'

People in their loops may appear to be 'a complainer,' or someone who enjoys painting themselves as the 'victim.' They may have strong negative preconceptions about the gender they're attracted to, which they can back up with names, dates, and persuasive examples. As hard as it is to watch someone in their Torture Loops, it's sometimes even harder to have compassion for, or even recognize, our own. One thing is certain, what starts as a habit, over time becomes a physiological response.

Behavioral researchers at Stanford University in the 1970s first discovered that human beings would go out of their way to defend their innate biases, even *more so* when they were given contradicting proof. Once we form a theory, we will go to amazing lengths to collect evidence about said idea to keep proving that it's true. Apparently, we want to be right so badly, even our brains cling to false information to prove a point.

Once subjects in this particular 'confirmation bias' study were told the original evidence fed to them was a lie, they went to *even further* lengths to defend that same belief. This is also referred to as cognitive distortion or cognitive dissonance. Perhaps the original idea has now formed its own Loop and the brain learns to hold onto that that pattern. Maybe we humans are just stubborn motherfuckers.

So why would we hold onto opinions that are so clearly not serving us, when it comes to something as awesome as fucking? Over time even awful notions we've internalized like "I'm a piece of shit" become comfortable because they can help us avoid things we don't want to look at. They feel good, in a self-righteous sort of way, "Haha, told you I was a piece of shit." If I'm a piece of shit, I don't have to take responsibility for my behavior, I can just wallow in my shittiness for all eternity. It's just not as sexy as is sounds...

So how do we break out of the Torture Loops that stop us from getting laid? For a start, substitute whatever you think right now with the knowledge that YOU WILL GET LAID. Of course, you will. *Why not you?* In the coming chapters you will learn how unseen prejudices and ideas have stopped you from getting your needs met, especially in a subject as touchy as boning. (Don't worry, I didn't forget about boning.)

1.5: Needs vs. Wants

Years ago, when my storybook marriage unraveled, friends and family looked on aghast. How could I create this disaster just to meet some kind of imagined 'needs?' The truth was by the end of my marriage, while my *wants* were indulged, my *needs* were ignored, and this was why I was blisteringly unhappy. The deeply satisfying, passionate life of my dreams was waiting, as soon as I was willing to stop treating something I *needed* for fulfillment, as just something I *wanted*.

Like many other women in certain enclaves, I spent years burying my true instincts under select items from Louis Vuitton. Even though I lost decades-long friends and in the small community where I lived it was as if a scarlet letter was emblazoned on my chest, being the 'town whore' for simply leaving my husband was, in retrospect, a small price to pay. (You say town whore like it's a bad thing.)

In the context of sex, a *want* is a whim or a temporary caprice that may or may not involve one or more mechanical acts. A *need,* on the other hand, is what underlies those wants, and drives us towards getting them. As I tell my

Sexual Intuitive® clients multiple times a day, "We do not argue with our own needs, we find ways to meet them."

Fulfilling a sexual need is like finding that miraculous extendable back scratcher to reach that one part you can't otherwise get to. The result is a heavenly, "Ah...that's better." Finding someone to do that to, with, and for, is the ultimate bliss. It is what I intend for you, and what you will magnetize once you know more about where your own itches are located.

Knowing what your needs are also prepares you to understand how to meet someone else's, making you, at the very least, an exceptionally desirable bedmate. This is different than projecting on someone what you think their needs are ('I can't wait to make you cum 100 times with my mouth') by assuming that just because you're into something, they will be too. The more curious you are about someone's actual groove, the more specific you can be about where exactly your tongue fits, so to speak.

A need is also different than a desire. Like maybe you really *want* a blowjob right now, but you don't technically *need* one. At some point, if you're in a relationship with someone, and the energy has become unbalanced between you, you may legit *need* to have your dick sucked to restore the balance of energy in the relationship. Obviously, this doesn't mean that the person you're dating *owes* you a blowjob, but it does present the opportunity to communicate about why they only want to do that on your birthday.

I hear a similar corresponding complaint from a lot of my female clients, "Why won't he/she/they go down on me?" Perhaps these vulva-owners are just seeking to fulfill the underlying need for sexual intimacy, but maybe they're not. If they're indeed looking for intimacy, it may be that being licked, sucked, and eaten is the only way to fulfill that need at the present time. From my coaching experience I know that anyone can reach a point when a passing desire becomes a need— when it cannot wait any longer, when you're so hungry for it you become bitter, angry, or otherwise unwell.

The idea of understanding your needs in the context of a more casual encounter is to pick people who won't leave you perpetually disappointed. In a relationship, this awareness can head off resentment before it gets to the point of being irreparable. The more you work on understanding how to scratch as many of your own itches as possible, the more freely you can turn to someone else to finish the job.

Part of admitting who you are is realizing there are some itches you can't scratch for yourself. One of the most toxic ideas prevalent in the self-help movement is 'You have to love yourself before you can love anybody else, or be loved.' Bullshit.

Let me once and for all disprove the theory that you have to be perfectly conventionally attractive, perfectly emotionally stable, or perfectly *anything* to get and keep a great sexual relationship. You don't have to wait until you're 'perfected' to have an equally imperfect person see the wonderful, unexpected charm that makes you hot in your own unique way.

Question anyone who tells you, "You have to be your own cake; someone else can only be the frosting." Relationships, even one-night relationships, are far more complicated than that. Who cares if you're the cherry or the frosting or the motherfucking fondant? What matters is we're all made of the same gooey, fleshy ingredients, and together we make a damn tasty concoction.

When we deny our own needs or have them ignored by someone else, we move further into inauthenticity, away from our true selves, and into emotional distress. This kind of continued stress can exacerbate or trigger existing tendencies towards mental illness. I'm not suggesting that mental illness occurs because of sexual repression, and if you know you're clinically depressed or anxious please do all you can to get treatment—therapy, natural remedies, medication—whatever works. I'm just asking you to consider that if you weren't getting your needs met, *of course you would be depressed.* In the next chapter, you'll start to identify and validate your basic needs, so that you can go about getting them met, as well as becoming the kind of person who can meet others' needs, not just on their birthday...

1.6: Identifying Your Needs

The following are some examples of basic needs you might identify for yourself. For each one I include a DIY section, so you can work on meeting these needs for yourself whether or not a potential partner has space on their 'dance card.' *Remember that fulfilling our own needs is not a prerequisite to getting laid.* It's just an ongoing approach to finding a partner from a place of abundance, instead of starvation. See which of the following core needs resonate for you:

Touch: After the fall of communism in Romania, the world was shocked to discover orphanages where children had been left without human touch, and as a result had a catastrophic failure to thrive. This neglect caused anxiety, depression, and other mood symptoms, even resulting in slow brain development and low IQ. Skin contact and physical affection are still *essential* for many in adulthood, as specified in the *Five Love Languages* by Gary Chapman, ensuring that the love you're expressing towards your partner will actually be 'felt' by them.

DIY: When your skin hungers for touch, it's also a need you can get met outside of sex. Hug a (consenting) family member, or go to a 'cuddle party' in your city. Get a massage or some bodywork; by all means get some hand relief (i.e. a happy ending) if you can find it legally where you live. Hug and stroke yourself. Touch is not some kind of luxury item you can't afford, it's a staple. No one can dictate how much touch is the right amount for you, and you can set an intention to find a corresponding Affection Slut.

Safety: It's perfectly fine to need safety as a prerequisite to getting sexy with a potential partner, or a current partner. *It is your responsibility to protect your own safety, with your actions, words, and habits.* While this is not always possible, because some events are completely unpredictable, what you can control is committing to your own safety as a need, and not accepting anything less. (Throughout the course of this book, you will become attuned enough to your gut instinct to stop seeing a bunch of red flags as a parade.)

Feeling safe can be especially crucial for women, people of color, trans folks, or anyone who has been traumatized by abuse. If you don't have any sexual or other trauma, or were privileged enough to have grown up in an environment where you felt mostly safe on both a physical and interpersonal level, it can be hard to understand why someone who hasn't had the same experiences might require safety as the bottom line of any dating interaction. Respect when someone is forthright and brave enough to communicate a boundary or safety requirement by honoring it. If you believe they're overreacting or being paranoid, do some homework—either culturally or with a specific intention to understand their needs—instead of accusing them of overreacting or being paranoid. The bonus is that the person you're attracted to will feel safe enough to be their natural, filthy selves in your presence!

DIY: *I will address more about safety in the last chapter in this section entitled Fuck Trauma, but there are many good shortcuts to soothing yourself if your body is feeling threatened by something that is not an actual threat. Proprioceptive input (sensations from joints, muscles and connective tissues) can be very comforting, and you can get it by lifting, pushing, and pulling heavy objects, such as by lifting weights or bracing and pushing into a wall. Even wrapping yourself in a weighted blanket, or strategically using sandbags or weights on different places of the body can provide containment. An old hypnotherapy trick is to write the word 'safe' or 'calm' on your thigh with your finger.*

Being seen: A great erotic encounter can help you feel seen, heard, noticed, and understood in an entirely different way than anything else, and therefore has great healing potential. When someone truly empathizes with you, it's not only healing, but can be super arousing, as they intuitively pick up where they will take things next. You might have other tenets that are important to you in life and relationships like Communication, Self-expression, or Attention, but the underlying need driving these is still *Being Seen*.

DIY: *The more you work on paying attention to how you operate, the more someone else will complement what you already have, as opposed to feeling pressure to provide a 'center' for you. You can put your energy in other areas besides sex, such as your career, friendships, and creative outlets to gain validation. You can even use social media as a positive affirmation, as long as you're focused on communicating your truth, not on how many likes you should get for that truth.*

Sexual intimacy/connection: In the 1950s the sociologist Abraham Maslow composed a 'basic needs' pyramid, that featured both sex and sexual intimacy alongside food, shelter, and what we traditionally think of as sustenance. It *is* possible to experience sexual intimacy with someone even if you don't do anything sexy with them (see emotional affairs or platonic friendships). Also, not everyone feels intimate with someone just because they fuck; in fact many seek out encounters precisely because they don't feel intimate in the traditional sense.

If you recognize that you have a prerequisite for intimacy in order for a sexual encounter to be worthwhile, you have to be honest with yourself about that. That way you can pick partners capable of the kind of connection you're looking for. You can also make it clear to a potential partner that a truck stop bathroom hook-up is not your idea of heaven, unless of course the person is willing to make eye contact in the truck stop bathroom mirror.

DIY: *A good place to start is to work on building sexual intimacy with yourself, both physically and emotionally. That's why stroking yourself in sensual ways, whether to climax or not, is so good for you, especially if you do it as part of an ongoing fact-finding mission about how your own desire works. Even if the wildest thing you ever do in bed is leave the lights on, noticing which dynamics excite you is how you build familiarity/intimacy with what it is about getting laid that's essential for you. I will cover this in detail in the upcoming chapter Fuck Energy, but for now be open! If you discover in your exploration that for example, being turned into a sissy or a fuckhole is what you need, you don't have to waste time questioning the validity of that. Simply find communities of like-minded souls where you can get humiliated or used to your heart's content!*

Self-sufficiency/autonomy: Sociologists, psychologists, behaviorists and motivational experts have touted the need for autonomy as essential to human happiness. Only you can discern how independent you need to be to feel content. If you seek to be somewhat dependent on another, it is useful to start thinking about to what extent, reducing the problems caused by mismatched expectations. You can fulfill your need for autonomy by giving yourself the *gift of agency* when it comes to getting laid—in the last chapter I will cover how to get what you need on your own terms.

> *DIY: Only you can discern how much time and space you need to allow your own thoughts and feelings to percolate. No one has the right to take away your ability to take care of yourself, even with solitude, if that is a core need for you. You can commit to maintaining your independence, even once you find someone who rocks your world.*

BDSM: Do you already know or suspect that some part of the umbrella acronym for Bondage/Discipline, Dominance/submission, Sadism/Masochism might be for you? Consider that for someone hardwired towards BDSM it is in your DNA, and not partaking in it is akin to not taking insulin for a diabetic in that it results in sickness. In the case of BDSM, it's the 'sickness' that leads to wellness!

60

Dominance and/or submission could be basic needs for you, even if you don't commit a 24/7 BDSM lifestyle (unless you do!).

These tendencies are entirely individual and don't have to conform to gender stereotypes fed to us by popular culture. Not every dude craves being a Dominant machine ramming someone into oblivion, and while some women might enjoy a man 'taking charge,' it doesn't mean they want to be locked into a submissive role. You don't have to identify as any gender at all to know that elements of BDSM excite you. People don't necessarily need to be a 'Top' or a 'Bottom' all the time, or may fluctuate depending on whom they're playing with. How true is this for you?

DIY: Tying yourself up (self-bondage) or giving yourself discipline is very different than self-harming because it is structured and administered with love. You're looking to create the influx of the pleasurable endorphins you might get from pain, without the guilt or trauma that often accompanies self-harming. Keep in mind that self-bondage can be wonderful, but is also super dangerous, even for advanced practitioners. Educate yourself thoroughly before attempting any of this at home, in the same way you would when negotiating how you allow someone else to play with you. The potential for physical injury or emotional fallout is so great that these practices should not be undertaken lightly. Make sure you institute fail-safe protocols so you're not the only one who can get you out of a potentially sticky situation. Another way to DIY BDSM is to pay an experienced Dominatrix, Dominant, or submissive, either in their own dungeon or at a BDSM club, to give you what you lack, making you less likely to throw yourself at un-vetted candidates.

Taking Care of Someone/Being Taken Care of: If you have a yearning to take care of someone, you can choose to seek out a traditional relationship that has a nurturing quality. If nurturing is something that arouses you, you could also find someone to be your 'baby' or your protégé(e) as well as lover or friend. In the context of BDSM, you can meet these needs in a Mommy/Daddy relationship, or outside of BDSM in a 'sugar' type arrangement, when one person helps another financially in exchange for previously agreed companionship or other services.

A 'sugarbaby' may not conform to more traditional ideas of a 'partner you can take to Christmas dinner,' but can be satisfying if caretaking (giving or getting) stokes your erotic fire.

DIY: *Sometimes it can be hard to remember to take care of ourselves physically, spiritually, and emotionally. Daily rituals, even around the basics of hygiene, when done in a more intentional way can create an ambiance of self-care. Even taking a walk when you know you need to be outside (weather permitting) can be an act of taking care of getting oxygen flowing through your body (if you get around in a chair or scooter, hopefully you have access to being able to move outdoors as well). You might have the resources to pay someone to take care of you in a non-sexual way such as with different kinds of bodywork, beauty or other treatments, personal training, or yoga classes.*

Taking care of yourself emotionally might mean spending time with family, friends, or people who feel good to be around. Spiritual self-care could entail attending a church, temple, spiritual community, or creating some kind of private communion. Taking excellent care of yourself is good practice for taking care of another, even for one night, if you recognize that this is their need. You can also get a pet to take care of (by this I mean an animal pet, not necessarily a human 'pet' in the BDSM sense, though if you know you want to be someone's 'pet' or find a 'pet' of your own, you can work on joining communities where this is as natural and normal as breathing).

Family: Many people want to have a family but see it as something that will happen on its own eventually at some indefinable point in the future, when they are 'ready,' or as something they have already 'missed.' Knowing that you want some iteration of a family doesn't have to mean in some distant reality with one partner and a white picket fence, you can create an intention to have polyamorous relationships, a poly triad or 'pod,' choosing to raise children in this configuration, or not. Don't discount the fact that you have so many choices, and if you need a 'family' to feel whole, you can define what that looks like, based on what works for you.

Even if you don't feel ready to have a family at this moment in time, you could choose to treat your sexual experiences as part of a continuum towards that end, rather than a compartmentalized period of 'playing around' until you're ready to 'settle down.' (It's also okay not to have a need for family.)

DIY: Rather than desperately scrolling through Grindr for a life partner to start a family with, in the meantime you can intentionally form a community that acts as a 'chosen family,' perhaps one that is more validating than your blood relatives when it comes to getting your sexual needs met. This creates a nurturing environment where the seeds of getting laid will grow, rather than being shut down by people who might mean well, but exist within the confines of their own prejudices. Your Uncle Larry who hasn't had sex with Aunt Jill in a decade and thinks men who wear pink are 'homos' is probably not the place to bring your burgeoning sexual exploration.

Fetishes: Most people mistakenly believe that a fetish is in the category of a want—some fad that you can take or leave—but it is, in fact, a need. A fetish is the only way to access a singular place inside you that will fester and rot if left unattended. Even once you discover or admit what your fetish(es) may be, the road to self-actualization is not supposed to be linear, and in its very messiness lays the fun.

You don't have to be a self-identified 'deviant' to benefit from understanding your needs. If you do find out you're pervier than you thought, Google will quickly disabuse you of the idea that you are the only one, as well as providing places to experience feet, fangs, or filthy mommies. A judicious use of the back page of certain publications will unearth individuals who are into the same 'weird' shit you are!

DIY: There are plenty of places on the internet where you can quench a fetish visually, with images or 'camming.' The most important work to do is not to judge your predilections as 'fucked up,' but to figure out ways to meet the need in a safe way that doesn't harm others. If you're convinced your kink is 'impossible to achieve IRL', as long as it's consensual, your DIY work is to unearth the Torture Loops that present that impossibility as 'truth.' Don't listen to 'experts' that want to classify your special paraphilia as a 'disorder.' Hiring someone who is skilled in your fetish can be a great start to finding a willing participant either thrilled to engage because they have a complementary fetish, or down to negotiate a way for you to get your needs met that they're also comfortable with. Pro-tip: If you know you have a specific hankering that some might find off-putting you have to be honest about it. Just don't unload all your kinks at someone as soon as you meet them, leave a little time and space for things to unfold. Unless you met on peedrinking.com, it might be wise to save that tidbit until after desert.

To recap, your needs might include:
- **Touch**
- **Safety**
- **Being seen**
- **Sexual intimacy/connection**
- **Self-sufficiency/autonomy**
- **BDSM**

- Taking care of someone/being taken care of
- Family
- Fetishes

Other possible essential needs:
- Adventure/excitement
- Decadence
- Security (emotional or financial)
- Laughter
- Serenity/calm
- Sobriety (drugs, alcohol, other addictions)
- Predictability
- Consistency
- Respect
- Commitment
- Being Cherished
- Freedom (poly, swinging, or other kinds of monagamish relationships)
- Fuck Motivation (more about this in the next chapter)

In each case, you can follow the rubric above to see how you might fulfill these for yourself. By the end of this book, once your Sexual Intuition awakens, you'll develop an antenna for people who have dovetailing needs, and find yourself choosing each other effortlessly.

DIY: Now that you have some examples, write out the needs that resonated for you. I encourage you to list just your top 10, because these are at your core. Remember to try and boil it down to the basic need that is driving the desire, the place where if you keep asking, "Why do I need that?" the answer is "Because it's something I can't do without."

Of course, feel free to add others that are not on my list:

My Needs

1.
2.
3.
4.
5.
6.
7.
8.
9.
10.

Listing your needs is different to writing out desired character traits in a bedmate that put the emphasis on a list of 'criteria' that are supposed to provide you with a feeling of wholeness. The 'wish list' approach actually takes away your power, because you're waiting for someone else to be a certain way, before you can be okay. Know that you are okay, right now, exactly the way you are. In the next section of this book, you will learn how to source a feeling of being okay in your own body, and you may wish to return to your list with what you discover.

1.7: Fuck Motivated

Some people are strongly motivated by sex. They base their big life decisions on how to get some, get more, or get something hotter. Of course, sex is not something you 'get' from someone, it's something you *share* with someone, but sometimes it feels like you can only have the luxury of thinking that way when you're getting some.

Traditionally it was assumed that women have sex for love, and men put up with love for sex. In my experience, none of it has much to do with gender, but rather with the degree to which you are Fuck Motivated; that is, the kind of person for whom being able to get laid regularly and well is a high priority. In the past, this was called 'having a high sex drive' if you were a man. For a woman, it was called 'being a slut.'

I've known many Fuck Motivated women. We are sluts and we don't care if you think so. We will drive for dick, and we do not need you to market your penis to us (that's why a dick pic is not good marketing, but more about this later). Obviously, we will also drive for pussy, or for sexual benefits that have nothing to do with genital configuration. Paradoxically, many of us find that we can be sluts and also monogamous. Just because someone is Fuck Motivated, doesn't make them untrustworthy. In fact, you can absolutely rely on them to show up for a fuck-appointment.

Emily Nagoski, sexologist and author of *Come As You Are: The Surprising New Science That Will Transform Your Sex Life* describes two categories of people in relationships, neither of which fall along gender lines. You can be either the kind of person whose stress is *relieved* by sex, or someone who is *not in the mood* for sex when you're stressed. Stress can radically "throw on the brakes" to your sexual responses, to the point where you don't even feel horny. Think about what makes you less Fuck Motivated? Did you lose your Fuck Motivation after something specific that took place?

Maybe you feel like you used to be Fuck Motivated when it came to dating, but it went the way of your Fuck Mojo—south. Barring any hormonal or medical reasons, there's a perfectly rational explanation for why you may have given up on making sex a priority, even if you really, really like doing it.

Since the 1970's, Professors Edward Deci, Richard Ryan, and later Marylène Gagné PhD have studied how people motivate themselves to achieve goals. They called it Self-determination Theory (SDT) and found that the two broad categories to motivation were 'intrinsic (internally motivated) or 'extrinsic' (based on the possibility of outside goodies.) If you tend to be more *externally* motivated, and you haven't been laid in a while, *it's perfectly understandable that you might give up trying.* Without external validation, it would be like promising yourself pizza after a workout, and then every time you go to collect your delicious reward, the store is closed. Eventually, you might get frustrated enough to give up working out entirely, because where the hell is the melted cheese?

Understandably when it comes to a person or people rejecting you, it's easy to take it personally and even assume that one closed door means no pizza for you, *ever again.* At the end of this chapter, I've included constructive, positive steps to take to complete a break-up in a way that doesn't require the pizza you're no longer with to participate and leaves you free to move forward to find more pie!

Studies among millennials show they're having sex less and put sex as a lower priority when it comes to finding a mate. Of course, there is nothing wrong with choosing to have periods where it doesn't feel as urgent to get laid, or if sex is really not someone's thing. Where this is problematic is if choosing not to make healthy sex a priority comes out of a resignation that 'It's too hard' or 'You can't have it all.' I ask you, how have far have we gone wrong as a society, if the youngs don't want to fuck?

There's a reason why sociologist Maslow includes sex in that 'basic human needs' pyramid, and it is not just because it's literally essential to humanity's survival. Even if you're not having sex to procreate, the fuck instinct remains. One way to embrace that is to find a more *internal* source of motivation, one that can take you through the lean times.

To be internally Fuck Motivated is to connect to those sexual urges you allowed full expression in the previous chapter. If you have a vivid, dynamic, sensual relationship with your own desires, you can use it as the **engine** that drives you forward, up and out of insecurity. Most importantly, *you can learn to feed yourself* with fantasies, masturbation, reading and watching erotic material. In the previous chapter, we learned specific ways to keep yourself sufficiently satiated to approach getting laid with more levelheadedness.

If you're paying attention, you can immediately tell whether someone is Fuck Motivated when you meet them. An online dating profile will usually reveal it in the first sentence, and if not, there's always a little section that explicitly states whether they're looking for a relationship or a hook-up. Just don't expect that you're going to 'change someone's mind.' Not everyone is correspondingly Fuck Motivated at the time you meet them, and they're allowed to be on their own journey. If someone is not interested, trying to badger them, or steamrolling their consent is akin to standing outside a closed restaurant, banging on the door, ranting about damn restaurateurs *withholding* their pies. (You don't want to be that guy.)

Being willing to put in effort to get (and keep) a great sexual relationship is an underrated character trait. If you're Fuck Motivated it means you're proactive and realistic about rejection. The risk of rejection can be part of what makes the whole endeavor thrilling, because it means you have some skin in the game (literally). Getting rejected is not the time to say, *"I'm not going to give up on making this person fuck me."* That's not motivation, it's something else. If you're going to stand outside someone's window with a boombox blasting "In Your Eyes," only try that *once*.

Being Fuck Motivated is an ongoing 'can do' attitude, not contingent on getting affirmation from every single person you find attractive. It's having a strong enough center that it won't be shaken by some inconvenience or even awkwardness, because sex can be a little awkward and that's okay too.

You have to be honest about how Fuck Motivated you are at the present time, without berating yourself for it. If you're not willing to inconvenience yourself to get laid, this will most certainly get in the way of getting laid, but that's just your reality for today, and doesn't have to form another Torture Loop.

Many of us have the Bandwidth Issue, a limited capacity to take in more information or expend energy outside of survival, which we sometimes think precludes us from getting laid. In actuality that just might mean our dials are full for that particular day, not necessarily that we have to swear off dating entirely until all our ducks are in a row. Where the fuck are these ducks and who's to say what order they have to be in? In the next section of this book, you'll discover a new, more resilient foundation for Fuck Motivation, one that emanates from the endless source of your own Sexual Intuition.

DIY: The way to get over a crush/ex/divorce is to make a radical choice to forgive and move on. Burn some effigies. Say some incantations and shit. Hit a punching bag. Do whatever it takes to physically process any sadness, rage, frustration, or pain that is lurking in your body. In addition, write a letter to each one of the past crushes/lovers/spouses that still has some kind of hold on you. In this letter it is important that you:

> 1. *Express how the person made you feel, both good and bad.*
> 2. *Own up to your part in why things went wrong.*
> 3. *Offer something positive (such as your forgiveness or your good wishes).*

You may never send this letter (most of the time I recommend that you don't) so make it raw, honest, and colorful, as it is for you. Dare to expose yourself completely, then burn that fucker (the letter, not the person) together with the specters of past defeat. Excelsior!

Part 2.0: Uncovering Your Sexual Intuition

2.1: What is Intuition?

Time Magazine reports that in 2014, the U.S. embarked on a 4 year, 3.85 million dollar investigative study into how intuition can be used in combat. In the Vietnam War, Officer Joe McMoneagle used his legendary sixth sense to avoid unseen danger. In 2006, field reports from Iraq confirmed that Staff Sergeant Martin Richburg, using intuition, prevented carnage in an IED incident. If the U.S. military believes we can harness this powerful 'spidey sense' to *cheat death*, surely it can help us get laid?

For some, the word 'intuition' is loaded—try substituting 'raw instincts,' 'inner compass,' or even 'just knowing.' For the military too, the languaging has moved away from Extra Sensory Perception, or ESP, to being called 'sensemaking.' This is described in Department of Defense literature as, "a motivated continuous effort to understand connections (which can be among people, places, and events) in order to anticipate their trajectories and act effectively." In layperson's terms, this just means being able to take in the facts and then see *beyond* them to a deeper truth.

If you've ever 'just known' the right course of action, even when all signs said otherwise, you've already benefited from the extraordinary gift of intuition. If you take an honest look at your life up to this point, you'll see how seemingly random choices like picking one school over another, moving to another state or country, or 'running into' people you end up hooking up with, have brought you unexpected joy.

However, you may also have learned to distrust your 'sixth sense' because of two seemingly logical reasons.

The first is that most of us have suffered some form of heartbreak in our lives. Even if you're not an across the board Emotional, it's likely that at some point, you got wildly hurt. Congratulations! You took a risk, it got messy, and your heart got smashed to smithereens. This is a positive sign that you were playing on the court of life, instead of observing the action from the stands.

Even for emotionally balanced people, break-ups can feel fatal. For those with trauma, they can literally be so. For some, a heartbreak or loss of loved one(s) can pose the risk of suicide or even the lesser known Takotsubo or 'broken heart' syndrome, where a grieving person develops sudden cardiomyopathy. Emotional pain, while awful to endure, can be the worthwhile price we pay for allowing ourselves to get close to people.

In the intuitive sense, there are no 'mistakes.' When you assume your 'intuition' guided you to 'the wrong person' or 'the wrong experience,' how can you ever trust it again? There's no wrong person or wrong situation, there's only *what happened*. If you can separate 'what happened,' from what *you think* happened, you can recalibrate your intuitive compass going forward.

It's important to note here that your intuition, powerful as it is, does not qualify as 'implied consent.' When you find someone attractive, and your instincts tell you they feel the same way, verbal consent is the only way to confirm your instincts are correct, or that this means they even want to engage in sexy times with you. There are creative ways to check-in with someone to get consent throughout a date, but keep in mind your potential bedmate may also be reticent to communicate because of their own negative experiences with putting the brakes on a relationship or encounter. This is where it becomes so important to be able to read not only verbal, but non-verbal signals. If people had tails, they could wag to let us know when we're on the right track. I promise you that if you get adept at what I'm about to teach you, a person's enthusiasm will be as obvious as a wagging tail.

The antidote to the climate of panic that has sprung up around the #metoo movement ("Can't a guy try to get laid anymore?") is to build up the muscle of your most natural intuitive ability—*noticing*. The more you *notice*, the more you're able to make those connections *implied* by what you notice. So many dating pitfalls and even sexual assaults could be avoided if people committed to *really paying attention*. Even a cursory check-in will reveal the instinctive fact, *"This person is not into this."* The Scarcity Torture Loop is the idea that if you don't coerce or even force this person into sex right now you'll never get laid again. It is the voice of fear, it is the voice of evil and, more to the point; it is lying.

A negative sexual experience can paralyze people into thinking they can no longer trust their own judgment. While there are some things you *couldn't have known* in the past, going forward you can harness the power of *noticing* to read physical, verbal, and emotional cues. That way rather than being in wishful thinking, you can observe what a person is *actually* showing you about who they are.

There are ill-intentioned people in the world, but this is no reason to shelve your instincts entirely, in fact even more reason to get in touch with them. That voice of your intuition gets louder and louder the more you use it, so you'll be able to trust it when it says, "I need to get out of this situation safely," or even, "I wonder how close this Applebee's bathroom is to the front door."

If you've had a hunch in the past that turned out to be 100% correct, it may be frustrating but useful to notice **that one moment** where you decided to ignore it. Sometimes when we have a feeling or a hunch about someone, unless it is 'provable,' we don't consider it valid. The fact is that if you catch a bad vibe, or even a 'knowing' that a person will never show up for you the way you want them to, you don't owe anyone an explanation, least of all yourself. Your intuition carries with it a responsibility to honor it, whether or not that hurts someone else's feelings.

The second reason people learn to question their intuitive sense is thinking they don't have enough experience to know what they're doing. Maybe you want to have more or better sex, but you haven't had that much. Maybe you feel like you weren't great at it, so what the fuck would a *newb* like you know anyway?

Well, you know a lot. In fact, experience can be the enemy of intuition, because it makes you approach the new as if it were just an extension of the old. When fucking becomes rote it's because people decide, *"Oh, I know what this is."* When you approach sex with the 'clean slate' of naiveté, it sets you free to have no idea where this particular encounter is going. You can create an improvisational good time based on what's happening to yourself and your lover *in the moment*. To that person, your newness is a gift.

In the Icelandic documentary *"InnSæi: The Power of Intuition,"* scientists in fields as diverse as marine biology, psychiatry, and business make a convincing case for intuition being the ultimate problem-solving tool. Left and right brain thinking on their own have not helped us, the experts contend, what is needed is a blend of both, in a way that is non-linear.

Harvard Business school professor and former CEO Bill George says, "At the highest level all decisions are intuitive." If you're more of a *Cerebral*, you've tried rationality when it comes to sex and love, and perhaps seen the limits of that approach. The old adage is not to apply logic to an illogical situation. As George says, "We're complex beings, we're mind, body, spirit. If we can't see inside ourselves, we can't see our greatest capabilities, and we can't let our own intuition flow."

When it comes to sex, it's useful and valuable to study up on how biology works not just in you, but the people you want to sex (go read up about the internal clitoris and prepare to have your mind blown) but just having the information is not enough. It's how you move *past* what you know and fearlessly into uncharted territory that make you an exciting bedmate.

Right at this moment your intuition may be causing some kind of havoc in your life. I love the Martin Luther King quote, "A riot is the language of the unheard." In addition to the political context of these words, when your soul's voice is rioting, it is because it's dying to be heard. Going through life listening to that voice is like having a superpower—

one you can develop without being bitten by a radioactive spider—you will begin to activate it in the following chapter.

2.2: Practical Exercises to Develop Your Sexual Intuition

So how do you know when something is an intuitive hit, as opposed to just a thought or belief? Intuition appears somatically, as a 'knowing' or something that operates *in your body.* You might feel a tingling sensation in the back of your neck, or your hair might stand on end. You will sense a confirmation of something you already suspected, and it will feel right in a way you can't explain. It will literally stop you in your tracks, or direct you towards a positive action. It will empower you to get where you didn't know you already wanted to go.

I know that I'm about to get into kind of woo-woo territory, but it is my assumption that everything in life happens the way it's meant to. There are many belief systems (including traditional religions) that rely on this kind of faith, and while you may be non-religious, atheist, or more science-based, I'm asking you to go with me, as we continue to explore some things that seem more 'out there.' In the intuitive realm it's important to remain open to unconventional concepts, because of the interesting possibilities they allow for.

If you believe that intuition is a function of getting quiet and listening for the Divine, or the light, or some other higher power, go with that! Similarly to your own concept of God/Goddess, intuition won't steer you towards something that's harmful to you in the long run. Growth opportunities maybe, but always in service of a greater good, even if it's one you don't yet understand. If someone you picked through Sexual Intuition ended up being kind of a bust, you can still count on the fact that you were supposed to have an experience with them, just not the kind you anticipated. This is where it becomes important to check whether what you think of as your intuition, isn't actually an opinion formed out of some kind of negative bias or that old chestnut, the Torture Loop.

Torture Loops are the greatest enemy of intuition because they cloud your ability to tune into the signs coming from your body, as you're stuck in your head. Many Torture Loops start off as one of the most innocuous, but actually dangerous things on earth, which is an Idea. A really good Idea is the last thing you want.

Here are some examples of great Ideas:

- All men are predators.
- Women are bitches/cunts.
- That's gay.
- Pussies smell/taste/are bad.
- Cum is gross.
- Sex is only for good-looking people.
- Sex is only for when you're in love.
- Sex is only good when it's casual.
- Sex is only good when...
- All women want to see my dick.
- People/men/women can't be trusted.
- Relationships never work out.
- Everyone hates me.
- Everyone loves me.
- Anyone who loves me must have something wrong with them.
- I'm a bad person.
- I'm a perfect person and the world just hasn't recognized my genius.
- Life should be fair.
- No one can be married and have great sex.
- People are liars.
- I'm going to die alone, genitals in hand, with my face eaten off by cats.
- It's my parents'/ex's/the government's fault I can't get laid.

It's only over time that seemingly reasonable Ideas turn into bonafide Torture Loops. Unfortunately by that point, the neurons, nerve cells, and tissues have organized into 'grooves' in the brain that will continue to run on the same tracks unless they're carefully redirected. When you hear yourself make a blanket generalization about a person or group it's likely to be rigid thinking, and the more you convince yourself of it, the more you limit what is possible for you, and for your interactions with that group (#notallclowns).

McGill University brain scientists liken the process of retaining memories and even learning new words to forming "paths through a forest." They contend, "As people keep taking the same route through a forest, they wear out a path in it. And the more people who take this path, the more deeply it's worn and the easier it becomes to follow. The same goes for our memories: the more we review them in our mind, the more deeply they are etched in our neural pathways."

Behold, for a new baby Torture Loop is born!

When an idea continues to loop merrily along the same track, like a skipping record player, it forces you into the same stunted (or even criminal) sexual behavior. It convinces you that you'll never get laid, or that the people you're interested in won't be interested in you, or that someone is your 'soulmate' when they have clearly stated that they're *not*. If you're paying attention in the present moment, you can trust that you will catch the unmistakable signs of interest, of possibility, of consent. You will perceive the wagging tail.

DIY: *Write a list of seven points that are TRUE about each of these subjects. If you don't relate to or have moved beyond any of the following gender classifications, feel free to leave them blank, but it can be interesting to see how they've influenced you. Include both positive and negative traits; what you're looking for are long-held secret thoughts you've carried, and haven't necessarily shared unless you had your guard down (or were drunk):*

MEN (ARE):

1.

2.

3.

4.

5.

6.

7.

WOMEN (ARE):
    1.
    2.
    3.
    4.
    5.
    6.
    7.

PEOPLE (ARE):
    1.
    2.
    3.
    4.
    5.
    6.
    7.

*How do you know when a perception you have is intuitive? If it feeds into one of the negative preconceptions you unearthed in this exercise, **it's probably not intuition**. It's fine if you think that all men suck, unless you have a preference for fucking men, in which case you might be SOL. Conversely if you know that, you can find creative ways to find dudes that want to be hate-fucked.*

If you have a need to fuck a particular person that feels like it might be self-destructive, I'm one of the few coaches that will encourage you to continue to engage in that until you intuitively know you're done. (Of course, practice safer sex so they don't leave you with an unwanted memento, as well as making sure your safety needs are met to the best of your abilities.) In my experience as both a sex coach and a human, anything other than letting that 'fat lady' sing it out 'til she's done, just starves her to death. This leaves the bloody carcass of the unresolved affair in your psyche forever, with too many unanswered questions you once had the opportunity to resolve. Don't quit before the miracle of losing interest in someone naturally.

DIY: *Now this is where it gets tricky. For the following list, it will come in handy if you're willing to dig in deeper beyond what you believe is true, about 'how you are.'*

I AM:
1.
2.
3.
4.
5.
6.
7.
8.
9.
10.

Okay, deep breath. Here's the challenge, and where it's time to move away from black-and-white thinking to find the intuition underneath.

If you have a mostly high opinion of yourself, then you have likely become used to blaming the gender that you want to fuck for a lack of getting laid. "It's not me, it must be them," is an idea that can turn toxic over time, in ways we see over and over again, especially in domestic violence and the sick loners who end up perpetrating desperate acts of terror.

"It's either *my* fault, or it's *their* fault," is not an intuitive response, because intuition doesn't deal in absolutes. It's always 'heuristic,' or the hypothesis we go with because it allows us to move forward. Here is the more nuanced view, 'It is not *you*, or *them*, sometimes it *just is.*'

You can't underestimate the importance of timing in life, especially when it comes to sex, dating, and relationships. (Also, clowns.) When you meet someone, even if you're wildly attracted to each other, if it's not the right time for either one of you because you're not ready, or one of you is married or recovering from a bizarre nuclear accident, or dozens of other factors, this is no-one's *fault*.

Much of what transpires in what we call physical reality is esoteric, based on contracts and energies that we cannot see. Even if your worldview is scientific, you know that there are many things in the natural world that cannot be explained. Is it the squirrel's fault it wasn't in heat when the other squirrel was? Should we mistrust that squirrel forever?

Of course humans are more sophisticated than squirrels, but when it comes to sex and love, we behave in ways that defy explanation, unless we factor in intuition. As Stella says in Tennessee Williams' *Streetcar Named Desire*, "There are things that happen between a man and a woman in the dark – that sort of make everything else seem – unimportant." (This also applies to men and men, women and women, and whatever gender-expansive combo feels right to you.)

While absolutes can seem comforting, they're not helpful when it comes to approaching a new person and a new situation, or even the same person, on a new day. You have many more choices than you believe, and once you believe that, your brain will believe it too, and start to allow a more intuitive (and possibly mellow) approach to life.

People call the space between black and white 'living in the gray' but I prefer to think of it as existing in the Technicolor. Only there can you learn to give others (and yourself) the benefit of nuance. And nuance is *hot*. Welcome to the first flickers of your Sexual Intuition.

DIY: *Here's another advanced exercise to unearth where your innate biases are stopping your intuitive gift from coming through. Once again, feel free to modify the genders in this next bit; we're just playing with stereotypes here to see what we learn. Ruminate for a moment on sexual experiences you've had or fantasized about having, and then answer intuitively (first thought, best thought, no wrong answer):*

SEX (IS):
   1.
   2.
   3.
   4.
   5.

A GOOD GIRL (IS):
   1.
   2.
   3.
   4.
   5.

A BAD GIRL (IS):
    1.
    2.
    3.
    4.
    5.

A BAD BOY (IS):
    6.
    7.
    8.
    9.
    10.

A GOOD BOY (IS):
    1.
    2.
    3.
    4.
    5.

Can you perceive where these views might have constricted you when it comes to getting your actual needs met? Alternately, that some of these might reflect valid and intuitive preferences about the kinds of people that tend to turn you on and that's perfectly okay? This is important because if you know you're attracted to, for example, more 'dangerous' people because they eschew conventional life choices in favor of 'living on the edge,' you don't have to quibble with that. Maybe it's a matter of letting your intuition guide you towards choosing a 'free spirit' who has traveled a lot, over someone who is currently incarcerated. (That said, if you're intuition is guiding you towards prison love, please have at it!)

2.3: Get Back In Your Body

Perhaps you feel like you're already in your body, because in literal terms, of course, where else could you be? Your sexual needs can only be understood if you're paying close attention to what's happening to you *somatically*. 'Somatic' means 'of the body.' If you're not *aware* of the sensations in your own body, there's no vehicle for the intuition to come in.

Sometimes people with disabilities, including those with invisible illnesses, have a *greater* sense of who we are beyond our physical skin sacks. If you live in a body where you experience numbness, paralysis, or have had limbs amputated, this certainly doesn't preclude you from enjoying sex. The folks I've met (and dated) that get around in chairs or scooters, or have some kind of autoimmune illness may be more intuitive because of the richness of their experience. What matters is not the degree of physical sensation you experience, but your *awareness* of it.

The practical technique I'll give you at the end of this chapter is one I have used to help clients return to experiencing themselves fully. It's adapted and modified from the ideas pioneered by German psychologist Christine Schenck in her book, *The Marriage of the Physical Body and the Energy Body*. This short, dense book changed my life. (Heads-up: I'm wading into more esoteric territory. Christine offers evidence to prove her ideas, I don't have time to do so here, so if you need proof, by all means read her book!)

Christine contends that each person has an Energy Body and a Physical Body, and they belong together, though many of us aren't aware of them as distinct from each other. If it helps, you can think of your Energy Body as 'the essence of *you*, that's separate from who you are physically.'

The skin is the natural boundary of both the Physical and Energy Body, but people who've had trauma or are used to disassociating from themselves for some other reason, don't have an awareness of being *grounded* within themselves in that way. (When I use the word grounded in this context, I don't mean grounded the way you would be as a punishment, or in baseball, but being able to operate in the world from a centered, connected, reality-based place.)

Someone can be Physical Body dominant, when they're primarily concerned with the realities of the physical world; what's for dinner, where's the rent check coming from, how's the surf today? Energy Body dominant people are more about soul concepts, big ideas, philosophical questions—they want to float through life like a ball of energy and can find physical reality to be quite constraining. Which do you sense that you are? (You could be a mixture of both, with one being slightly dominant.)

One of my clients, Zeus, was suffering greatly with the anxiety he felt over his girlfriend. When they were actually together, Zeus felt mostly secure, and described their time together as "pretty much perfect." But as soon as he was away from her, the anxiety would begin. He's not a terribly jealous person, or generally insecure, just a fairly traditional, monogamous guy. He didn't want to crowd or overwhelm this woman, but no matter how hard he tried not to, she felt stifled. She used the rather odd words, "I feel like I can never miss you, because *you're always there.*"

Zeus and his girl only saw each other a maximum of three times a week, so on the physical plane they were not nearly *always* together. Much has been written about energetic cords that I won't go into here, but when I asked him to visualize the connection with his girlfriend his first instinct was of an electrical cord. And when I asked him whether it was connected to her head, her heart, or her pussy, he said the heart, on both her side and his. Then he confirmed what I already felt—the cord began in his chest, but when it connected into her, it was in the form of an electrical plug.

The day after I took Zeus through the exercise I'll share with you shortly, he sent me an email that said, "Thank you for changing my life." Within a week, his girlfriend began seeking out his company more, because she felt enough energetic separation from him to miss his presence.

These are difficult concepts to write about because they're more effective when felt experientially. When someone talks you through an exercise that returns your Energy Body to your Physical Body, you can have a profound and delicious sense of coming home to yourself. You're then available to be with people in a completely different way, whether you're fucking them or not. While it may be hard to describe, it's worth allowing yourself to imagine. One of the endless benefits of feeling more 'embodied' is seeing the difference in the way people respond to you.

Our Energy Body needs to be fascinated with the experience of staying in our Physical Body, but if this language is off-putting you can think of it as being like a potted plant that doesn't try to wander over into the adjoining pot, because it can only grow in its own soil.

The following exercise can open up a whole new way of life, if you let it. How you'll know you're in the sweet spot is that it will feel powerful and contained but maybe somewhat raw and vulnerable. Sometimes this rush of somatic awareness can leave you feeling somewhat bruised, but remember that your bruise might be someone else's permission to desire you.

DIY: Grounding Exercise for Sexual Intuition

Before we begin, set the intention for your Energy Body to come home to your Physical Body. If you feel numbed or unable to connect to certain parts of yourself, this can be worked on gently, energetically, and with time. Don't struggle.

Many people live up in their heads so it's usually not so difficult an assignment to be aware of that part of the body. The heart center, sex organs, and feet can be more challenging. Just notice, without judging. If you can, get someone you trust to read the grounding exercise to you, or even record yourself saying it and then listen. Get ready to save yourself...

Begin by sitting on a fairly hard surface, holding your back in a way that's comfortable but still straight enough to require some effort. Put your feet parallel on the floor, and rest your hands on your thighs. DO NOT CLOSE YOUR EYES. We want to have a sense of ourselves in physical reality, not float away. Find a gazing point, and with soft focus try to keep it the same for the entire exercise, though you can move it if you need to.

First feel your feet on the floor, beyond just the surface of the sole touching the floor or a sock or the inside of a shoe. Bring your awareness to the solidness inside your foot, without tripping out on the muscles or bones or tendons. You are simply noticing what's inside your feet. Now pay attention to the contents of both feet at the same time without moving or touching them.

Take your awareness up to your hips. Feel your buttocks pressing into the surface you're sitting on, and then move that awareness downwards to feel the solidness of your thighs from the inside. Then feel the insides of your knees, and the solidness between the calves and the shins, that connects into your ankles, and then down into your feet. You should now be able to have an awareness of your lower half grounded to the floor, and magnetized to the spinning core of the earth, but still located inside you.

Connect to your sex organs, and feel them from the inside. Can you feel all your sex organs, including your anus, without touching or moving them?

Now take your awareness up your belly across your chest or inside your breasts, and spread it out through your collarbones. Connect it from your lower back, to your mid-back, and spreading out to your shoulder blades. Feel the solidness of you in the

104

middle, and in the heart-center, where your Energy Body wants to be.

Breathe.

Feel your shoulders, and take the awareness down your arms to your elbows, and then down to your wrists, and sense the insides of your hands. Breathe, and connect the internal awareness of both your hands at the same time, both your feet at the same time, and your entire body from the neck down.

Now feel your neck, front and back, full and contained. And finally your head, your skull, and what's inside.

Feel your Energy Body completely inhabiting your Physical Body, and seal the deal by holding your own hand. This is what it means to 'show up for yourself.' This is being your own best friend through life. Believe the seemingly banal passing 'thoughts' you have at this time – they have been waiting to show themselves to you.

2.4: Fuck Energy

Now that you have a better awareness of cues from your physical body, I'm going to give you an intuitive tool used by pretty much everyone I've ever met who gets laid effortlessly. It's an ability that can be developed by anyone willing to drill down and be honest with themselves. I refer to it as being able to get in touch with your own unique Fuck Energy.

If you've ever stood next to someone in a private or public place and felt a rush of *something* coming from them, you've felt Fuck Energy. Some people call it *chemistry*, but I call it Fuck Energy because it doesn't actually have to involve another person. Your Fuck Energy lives in you all the time, someone or something—even a visual image—is just coming along to *awaken* it. (It's harder to have chemistry with yourself, though if you do, you probably take a lot of selfies.)

Those of us who have always felt the existence of 'energy' were treated like ninnies until the Great God Science—in the form of German physicist Dr. Fritz Albert-Popp—confirmed what intuitives have always known; all things animate and inanimate have a specific thermal reading and energy field in the form of tiny particles called 'biophoton emissions.' Just because science hasn't yet proven the existence of Fuck Energy, doesn't mean it doesn't exist.

Your Fuck Energy is as singular as a thumbprint, a living organism that continues to develop the more you allow it to. Undertake your Fuck Energy as a continuing research project—a fact-finding mission about both what *you're like* and *what you like* sexually—and it will continue to delight and surprise you. Sometimes that just means getting comfortable with whatever 'weird thing' you're into. I promise you, whatever it is; it's not *that* weird. In fact, usually it's either very common, or at the very least already has its own Fetlife.com sub-category.

Knowing how your own Fuck Energy functions is like unlocking the door to an intuitive way of perceiving both yourself and others based on being *really* comfortable with yourself. As sex educators we *love* encouraging you to masturbate, but the idea is to move on from unconsciously whacking it to something with a little more awareness.

This is where Mindful Masturbation comes in handy (ha). By age 21 many of us have masturbated for the prescribed 10,000 hours it takes to achieve mastery, but how many of us have done it mindfully, been more Buddhist about it, if you will? Sure, the Dalai Lama might not approve, but unless you're going to shave your head and wear one of those fetch vermillion robes, have a wank and Namaste.

> **DIY:** *For people with vulvas: Get a hand mirror to squat over or lie in front of to get familiar with your sex organs beyond a vague 'down there.' A site I also recommend to clients is omgyes.com, to shine a light on preferences that may be hidden, sometimes simply because we have an 'innie' instead of an 'outie' (because the vagina is internal, as opposed to hangin' out like a cock). There are also internalized cultural ideas that teach us to see vaginas as something shameful.*

I don't judge porn from some moral high ground but getting too used to porn as the only way you can cum sets up a mental hardwire geared towards the same, sanitized version of fucking, over and over, with a possible stagnation in growth, development, and sincerity. When you start to tune into the Fuck

Energy that appeals to you about a clip or image, you can use that to inform a real-time experience with a bonafide human, as opposed to trying to emulate what it 'looked like.'

A lot of porn is not made ethically, which besides the conscience factor, can make it difficult to read the Fuck Energy and figure out who is actually doing what to whom. Seek out some 'slow' porn, preferably with people who haven't been exploited making it, just like the slow food movement is designed to make you savor things, not just gulp it down like a hog *like we all could*. Try the work of pornographer Erika Lust, kink.com, Tumblr sites such as *Lady Cheeky* and *Let Me Do This To You*, and read some Anais Nin or other erotica.

Is there a running theme with the kind of energy you identify with in the erotic material you read, watch, and think about? Whether or not you use visual stimuli, pay attention to *what* specifically arouses you, without trying to figure out the *why*. For example, notice who's in charge (Dominant) and who's being controlled, annihilated, conquered, or overwhelmed (submissive) and what those energies *feel* like, instead of what they *look* like. Can you *be with* that without judging it, knowing it may be part of the needs you identified earlier?

The more kinds of sexual expression you expose yourself to, the more deeply you'll understand your Fuck Energy and what will match with that, as opposed to 'an idea' of what a potential bed-mate should look like such as, "She has to be a blonde supermodel with big tits." There's only one Kate Upton, and regretfully she's not interested in you (or me). However, knowing what you like, even what you *secretly* like, ensures *you'll know it when you see it*, and be all fired up to go for someone who's a better fit for you than Kate Upton.

Being specific about the kind of sex you want means getting more real, especially if your ideas are based on porn. Mindlessly consuming junk porn might be part of your journey, but it's probably not going to advance your skills, and might also set you up for disappointment. Flesh jiggles and moves, people have smells and hair where you don't expect; the fun part is that real stuff that differentiates a live person from a hypothetical. It's finding out what Fuck Energy that excites you on that particular day.

I find it useful to think of sex as more than just a set of physical acts and more like a *pathway*. The actual *connection* doesn't take place in the physical—the mechanics of 'parts rubbing' are just a way to access mental, emotional, or energetic states. It's the same way athletes who do distance running don't necessarily do it for the muscle pain and broken toenails (unless they're masochists, which is a perfectly healthy way to get that need met) they do it to get the 'runner's high' (running IMHO is not as much fun as fucking).

Fuck Energy is what makes getting laid feel different with different people at different times, *even if the mechanical acts are the same.* It's also why the same acts can feel vastly different with the same person on different days, because it depends on where each person is energetically. (Of course, hormonal, mental, emotional, and physical circumstances play a part in this difference, but to perceive someone's Fuck Energy is to encompass all of these as a whole.)

If you're not intuitively in touch with your own Fuck Energy, it might show up as, "I'm just not that attracted to many people." If you're attracted to less people, your dating pool is smaller, so it's a good idea to get tuned in so you can get more turned on!

There are many other practices and activities that can tap you in to your Fuck Energy such as exercise, yoga, all types of dance, Tantra, and other Somatic-based sexuality workshops. Cannabis is becoming increasingly touted for its ability to lower inhibitions, as well as relax specific physical conditions that keep you from experiencing your own Fuck Energy (if it is legal in your State or country). Even MDMA aka Molly or ecstasy, or psychedelics like LSD, *ayahuasca* or mushrooms can help you tune in when taken in a safe environment. (I'm not telling you to take drugs, I'm just not telling you *not* to, unless you've chosen sobriety as a way of life, in which case stick with that.)

Being a person who's in touch with your own Fuck Energy is incredibly empowering, because most people aren't aware of themselves beyond the shallow, such as thinking they're hot, attractive, or fuckable, or conversely neither hot, attractive, nor fuckable. Trust me when I tell you, *everyone is fuckable*.

Every human being has others in the world whose Fuck Energy matches their own perfectly.

You may already have met some of them...

DIY: *Practice being next to people you may or may not be attracted to, and sensing instead of either staring, judging, or ignoring them based on a narrow set of physical traits. Learning how to sense someone's Fuck Energy is a better predictor for how good they're going to be in the sack with you anyway. Looking beyond the superficial is not called 'dropping your standards' it's called 'growing up out of middle school' and getting laid accordingly.*

2.5: How to Change Your Fuck Frequency

When it comes to sex, all people (even asexual or demisexual people) broadcast something about their sexual tastes and preferences, often without knowing it. This is their (and your) Fuck Frequency. I'm talking about Frequency like a radio frequency, as opposed to frequency like how often you do something. In this case, sensing another person's Fuck Frequency—as well as adjusting your own—will increase the frequency of your fucks.

When you practice being able to observe someone without objectifying them, you put aside *whatever you think you know about them* to allow your powerful intuition to kick in. As you learn to feel without touching, see without looking, and *perceive* with all your senses, revelations will appear that can only have come from your intuition. Also, as most people crave to be *seen,* they'll appreciate you being able to tune in to their Fuck Frequency, as opposed to being shoved into a box, even an adorable one marked *Cute Redheads.*

Actors observe people in everyday life and what they're telegraphing about their inner lives with tiny details. Noticing how a strap on a sundress is affixed with a safety pin instead of a button, for example, can be used it to intuit the truth of a character. They understand that subtle physical choices someone makes often broadcasts who they are, way beyond the verbal.

It behooves you to become *fascinated* by how people choose to express themselves—their mannerisms, habits, and behaviors—beyond their tits or their cars. What sexual signal are they emitting, if any? What can you learn from them? Can you postpone judging and evaluating them at least until you've checked in with your intuition, the one sense that might recognize their essence beneath the funky mustache? Becoming a person who notices these details in others not only makes you more perceptive, but also changes your own Fuck Frequency from 'Grasping' to 'Receiving.'

This practice takes away the mistaken belief that only someone else can make you sexually 'come alive;' that if you're not 'chosen' you have been judged as less than, and therefore are not entitled to feel desirable. This is why pretty much everyone hates dating, because it can feel like one of those carnival games where someone is dunked in water, or a Sex

Interview. The way the hetero culture particularly has evolved, women are societally still expected to be reticent about sex, while men are pursuing it. By being ignorant of a person's actual Fuck Frequency, we find ourselves stuffed into the straightjacket of traditional dating like some kind of generic, anxiety sausage.

An inability to pay attention to Fuck Frequency can also result in issues of consent being ignored. Due to culturally ingrained misconceptions, even a somewhat well-intentioned guy can assume that a woman has to be 'coaxed' into sex, unless she's a porn performer, sex worker, or someone who writes about sex on the internet in which case she's game for anything. (Ditto porn performers, sex workers, and sexuality bloggers/professionals of other genders.) All of these stereotypes are incredibly damaging.

Most adult women do not need to be coaxed into sex, because we are as horny as you are, or more so. If you're paying attention to someone's Fuck Frequency you can't miss the difference between someone who wants to be coaxed (for the percentage of the population that needs a 'coaxing' energy or gets aroused by it) and someone who genuinely doesn't want to sleep with you but may be trying to let you down easy. This is not the time to try to put in practice those great business webinar skills you learned that turn 'no's into 'yes's.

Someone may be reticent to tell you they're not interested because either it feels unsafe to do so, they have some other issue related to 'not wanting to hurt your feelings,' or many other scenarios like being your client, patient, or potential employee. However, if someone does tell you they're not DTF, at any point before, during, or after a sexual encounter, *believe them.* If in doubt, ask. Don't rely on what you believe a person's Fuck Frequency is telling you, without confirming it with them using actual words, letting them know that whatever they choose is okay with you. This also moves your dial over from 'Entitled to Get Laid Because I'm Horny' to 'Safe and Fun to Have Sex With.'

Conversely, if you have empirical evidence that the same kind of abusive humans are attracted to you over and over again, it may be worth looking at your Fuck Frequency. Are you too accommodating because you think you have to be? Are you dropping verbal and visual cues that your needs are not important? Are you looking for someone's approval, as opposed to investigating them as a pleasure-seeker on equal footing with you?

Throwing out mixed signals with words vs. actions is understandable because people (especially women, POC, and trans folks) are afraid of very real possible consequences that can happen if they assert themselves. However, changing your Fuck Frequency to 'Pleasure and Safety Cruise Director' is one way to magnetize people that treat you with respect.

You can't change your Fuck Frequency until you check out what you're unconsciously revealing to people. Ideally, your manner accurately reflects who you are at the present time. It's good to know when it's inappropriate to unleash your inner freak, unless you find yourself always holding back your truth because you don't want to make others uncomfortable. The more chill you are with your own Fuck Energy, the more authentically you will appear in the world; ergo, the sexier you'll be.

This is the opposite approach to one popularized by the dude who called himself *Mystery*, a Canadian 'pick-up artist' who used a somewhat 'queer' presentation (fluffy hat, eyeliner and nail polish) as well as various 'techniques' to pick up women. This approach was documented, then later discredited by the same writer, Neil Strauss in *The Game-Penetrating the Secret Society of Pick-up Artists.* According to pick-up culture, you had to 'pretend' to be someone other than you were to get laid, basically implying that you, as you were, were not sufficient, and that all women were drooling morons.

The most pernicious 'pick-up technique' of all was *negging*, trying to inflame someone's insecurities so they'll think you're their only option. Negging is still rife in dating, as my female clients can attest. My ears prick up when I hear of criticisms slyly inserted between compliments on dates, which just makes a chick think someone they might otherwise have slept with is kind of an asshole. It's the worst piece of dating advice you'll ever hear.

One reason negging is ineffective is that it restricts the other person being free to share their Fuck Energy with you, so it tunes their

Fuck Frequency to 'Cagey.' Women especially, as historically the more preyed upon gender, need to feel *safe* to unfurl their inner fuck monster. You have more finesse than that played-out shit, so develop a built in Fuck-Energy-ometer instead.

Taking ownership of your Fuck Frequency is actually about turning the dial *up* on your self-expression. There are people who want to fuck Trekkies that don't want to fuck dotcom billionaires, and they will find you because *they're already looking to find you*.

As I mentioned in the Identifying Needs chapter, everyone needs to look out for their own safety, and regardless of what happened in your past, it was not your fault if you were victimized. Going forward, it's important to respect what feels good to you, and what doesn't, and remember you don't owe anyone a pity encounter of any kind. You can be direct, forthright, and still be (where possible) kind, and this will actually change your Fuck Frequency from 'Prey' to 'Badass,' conveying a stronger message to predators to keep it moving. (I have a dream that if enough people do this, eventually predators will have no one to victimize, but this may not happen in my lifetime.)

If you're operating in an intuitive state, there is less of a chance that you will voluntarily put yourself in a dangerous situation because you'll be better able to *believe* your body about someone who feels 'off' to you. When you're on a date, or even meeting for 'not a date,' you don't have to focus on potential pitfalls as inevitable. The key is paying attention to *how it feels in your body to be next to someone,* because that's you'll feel their 'red flags' flapping in your gut.

You will sense when someone's Frequency doesn't match with yours, even if it contradicts the image they're working to present. If you're not sure, always meet in public, and institute whatever other safety protocols you need (screenshots, addresses, or text/phone safe call check-ins with trusted friends). Work on getting to know people better and intuiting clues between those hilarious cat anecdotes. The sharper your antenna (even if it's just a finely tuned bullshit detector) the more quickly you'll be able to accomplish this recon.

Being able to tune into a person's Fuck Frequency without pigeonholing them is important for everyone. For example, many men I've met and coached feel they're not seen beyond being some kind of 'dinner buyer' or Romance Bot who is expected to 'sweep a woman off her feet.' This is prevalent in older generations where there's an expectation of what it means to be a 'gentleman' and I will not get started here on how annoying and counterproductive this is. All people need to inquire deeply into themselves about any built-in expectations they have that are based on gender. If a guy buying you dinner makes you wet, that's very different to believing if he doesn't then he doesn't 'deserve' to get laid.

If more people made an effort to *really see* each other, there would be less gender-based misapprehensions that lead to harassment, assault, or worse. (For trans people it's especially important to be seen beyond a narrow set of preconceptions that put them at a greater risk for both stranger and intimate partner violence.) Remembering that someone's gender doesn't reflect what they're into increases the chances they'll want to do that thing with you.

Our electronic devices, sound-bytes, and hot takes have shrunk our attention spans. The most valuable tool you have in *getting* someone's attention is becoming someone who is *paying* attention. When we feel someone being receptive to us, we're more receptive to them, and anyone who ever 'picked up' anyone for a mutually satisfying experience did it because they were paying attention to Fuck Frequency, not because of some formula given to them by a man wearing a fluffy hat.

I practice the grounding exercise from earlier in this section many, many times a day, to refine my body's ability to communicate with me intuitively. When you're energetically in your body, you can begin to refine your Fuck Frequency to attract likeminded freaks, darlings, or freaky darlings. You are beginning to know what your *art* is, sexually speaking, and sexual sophistication is an underrated aphrodisiac. When you have a sense of what your Fuck Energy feels like, the idea is to let your Fuck Frequency reveal that. You are now ready to enter (dun dun dun) The Fuck Zone...

DIY: What Fuck Frequency do you broadcast? Take an inventory of what someone might see when they look at you. Do you take care of yourself like someone who cares for you? Does your life express who you really are, or are you in action about having a life you recognize as your own creation? Using movies, books, nature, and pop culture, have some fun both naming your Fuck Frequency, and considering what Frequencies you find attractive. Here are some examples:

- *Beatnik poet*
- *'Adrian' from Rocky*
- *Bladerunner*
- *Frightened spider*
- *Maggie Gyllenhaal's character in Secretary*
- *James Spader's character in Secretary*
- *Wood nymph*
- *Magenta from Rocky Horror*
- *One of the four Sex and the City women*
- *Winona Ryder*
- *A President immortalized on Mt. Rushmore*
- *Baltic Eurovision contestant*
- *Tom Bergeron*
- *Survivalist*
- *MILF*
- *Post-Apocalyptic Barbie*
- *A Tarot Card of your choice such as The Fool or Temperance*

You may want to ask friends about how they see you, and you might be surprised at how you come across. You can also sit in public places and check out people's Fuck Frequencies, this is not the same as gawking, you can even sense them with your peripheral vision. In this exercise, we're using celebrities, stereotypes, and icons to get you closer to the truth—your Fuck Frequency is entirely your own, beyond your physical attributes and deserves to be appreciated and reveled in. Remember, you're the only wood nymph of your kind.

2.6: The Fuck Zone

Have you ever experienced a time when things were *easy*? When you were 'in the zone,' 'in the flow,' or just plain in a good mood? In that state of being everything seems different, with almost an inevitable sense that things will go your way. When it comes to getting laid, I call this the Fuck Zone.

The Fuck Zone is the grid of sexual energy that percolates around us at all times; a state of heightened sensory awareness or aliveness where even the wind feels like a caress against your skin. Tapping into this place is not a matter of stepping into some kind of parallel universe or fantasy world where everything is perfect and everyone wants to fuck you. It's learning to use the power of the present moment to fully awaken your perception, both physical and intuitive. In the Fuck Zone, you take pleasure in even the simplest and most banal of things, deriving emotional and spiritual joy from your surroundings. The best part—it's available to you RIGHT NOW.

When you're in the Fuck Zone, you notice the ambient Fuck Energy that's already flying around. By the mere act of noticing it, you become someone other people notice. Being conscious and awake in this way sets you apart from the majority of humans who go through their lives on autopilot. Entering the Fuck Zone is an *ontological* change, i.e. a change in your *being.* This isn't about positive thinking but transforming the way you *exist* in the world. It opens up a world of enjoyment you may have previously cut off or ignored before you learned to harness your Sexual Intuition.

Here are five ways to put yourself in the Fuck Zone (aka the Fuck Matrix) right now:

1. **Meditate.** You can learn how to meditate with the use of an app (like Headspace) by taking a class, or looking at instructional videos online. In terms of the Fuck Zone, a state of present moment awareness means being able to respond to your environment, including people you're attracted to, in a relaxed and spontaneous way. It can help quell any anxiety that rises up in your body around sex or dating, or being 'up in your head' to establish a connection with someone you're interested in. George Mumford, the former athlete turned sports psychologist and meditation

coach to legends such as Michael Jordan, Kobe Bryant, and Shaq describes the state of being 'in the zone' as something that happens when "your conscious thinking is quiet and you let your body do what it does." (Mumford's athletes even recorded a '3-second time lapse between stimulus and response,' certainly enough time to wow someone with either your wit or your audacity to sit back and chill.)

2. **Flirt.** Flirting is not some kind of 'means to an end' —you don't have to go through with whatever your longing glances or teasing smile may convey. Rather, it's a way to tell someone, **"I see you."** To see and be seen is not the norm in a culture that demands we continually generate results at a breakneck pace. Pressing pause on 'business as usual' to pay special attention to another person's energy can make a life-changing difference to them, whether you ever see them again or not, let alone naked. Remember: **No-one owes you a response when you flirt with them, especially if they don't feel like being seen.** The more intuitive you become,

the more you'll know when to playfully speak what is unspoken and when to STFU and pay for your coffee.

3. **Develop gratitude.** Gratitude for what you have burns off anger at what you don't. Twelve-steppers sometimes have to learn to be thankful by losing everything, but you don't have to (if you already have congrats! You're even more equipped to take an honest inventory of what has and hasn't been working in your life thus far!) Even if you're crushed by a heartbreak or romantic failure, gratitude propels you from a starting line of abundance, as opposed to giving off a seeking-a-warm-body-to-distract-from-the-misery-of-life-with-myself vibe.

4. **Be turned on.** By everything. And everyone. Seeing the attractive qualities in every single person is so much more enriching than approaching them with a critical eye. Even inanimate objects like art, nature, or a flat tire can convey their own beauty. No one has to know about your erotic tire fetish if you don't want them to (ooh those sexy grooves and the

way they just *explode* on the highway), this is a matter of developing a talent for seeing the exquisite in the everyday. You can have a boner for life itself! Keep in mind if you're constantly horny this is not someone else's obligation to alleviate. However, if people and what you can offer them turn you on, they will be turned on by you.

5. **Reframe**. Dr. William Tiller, a bioenergetics physicist at Stanford University was able to prove (using fruit flies of all things) that our intentions have measurable effects on the physical realm. From Buddhists to Tony Robbins to Fox News, many have been able to use the knack of creating our own reality, whether or not it lines up with some kind of objective 'facts.' Most facts are subjective. It's your world, baby, we're all just living in it, so why not make it a

   juicy one?

Your Fuck Zone is the sweet spot where you're connected to your life's purpose, a state in which you can't help but attract fireflies to your light. It requires commitment and effort, but once you are used to functioning in this intuitive way, eventually it becomes the norm, and something you will want to sustain even after you're consistently getting laid. Here are the five most common issues that take you out of the Fuck Zone:

1. **Anger.** While I understand that nothing beats the excruciating hell of enforced celibacy, if your online dating profile or IRL persona leads with venting about mistakes perpetrated by others, you're in the Anger Zone, and no-one wants to visit there because it's *scary*. (The only way to be in the Fuck Zone and the Anger Zone simultaneously is when you're hate-fucking someone, but that's some next level shit we're not going into right now.)

2. **Benching Yourself.** When we close off to the grid it might be because of a million reasons that *seem* valid, but have nothing to do with how desirable we are like, "I've put on weight" or "I'm just waiting until I get my career on track." You can be on the court engaging with life and relationships even if you're not perfect yet, promise.

3. **Mental Health Issues.** The depression, anxiety, and myriad symptoms many of us endure keep us out of joy, and in survival mode. I understand deeply that sometimes shit don't feel that joyous (sic) and how it may feel like finding someone to fuck is too overwhelming or difficult. Why not use how much you want to get laid to motivate you to handle any unaddressed mental health issues? Think of all the wonderful dopamine, norepinephrine, and serotonin surges frequent sex makes available. By avoiding managing any mental health issues you may have, you may be fucking yourself in the bad way. On the other hand, learning how to navigate the world of sex and dating with a brain that is not neurotypical keeps you in the Fuck Zone because by definition it requires a superlative mastery of present moment awareness.

4. **Addictions.** Whether it's alcohol, cupcakes, or video games, your intuition already knows what your compulsions are costing you. Overindulging in your vices is not *morally* wrong. Instead of judging yourself harshly, consider how

finding an authentic sexual expression could be made more available by cleaning up your act.

5. **Monogamy.** Sometimes it can feel like if you're in a monogamous relationship, you have to stop engaging sensually with life because it feels 'cheaty.' In actual fact, you can be 'in the flow' enjoying people's attractiveness without necessarily telegraphing your availability or acting on your impulses. Instead, you can bring the FZ home where your partner might enjoy sharing life with someone who knows they don't own their partner's sexuality (unless it turns you on if they do, see: BDSM). There's no reason to give up enjoying the beauty of people just because you're presently choosing to be naked with only one of them. Worst case scenario, even if a relationship ends, you haven't made one other person the source of your entire experience of sexuality, and you don't have to go back out there beyond the Friend Zone, into the No Friend Zone. (Also, a relationship is *less* likely to end when partners feel free to

express perfectly normal attraction to others.)

I've intuitively felt this invisible Fuck Matrix across the more than twenty countries I've visited since I became sexually active, and maybe even before. Interestingly, I've never *not* felt it, except during two periods in my life. The first was when I was a 17-year-old fashion model attending Melbourne University. Despite already working in national TV commercials, print ads, and editorials, I was convinced I couldn't have *paid* a young horny college boy to fuck me (I now understand that this was related to projecting a Fuck Frequency of 'Scary.') The second dry spell was when I was married and expected my then-husband to be the source of my entire experience of sexuality.

When I left my marriage, I was suddenly aware of a whole other existence that I'd pushed beneath my radar. It was downright bizarre how the same physical reality seemed entirely different to me than it had even a month before. I would repeatedly friend (single) people that 'felt right' on social media based on a gut feeling and they would immediately message me and start something, even though I was no longer at the media-approved level of alleged youthful perkiness. (I'm not saying you should expect that this will work for you every time, I'm just reporting.)

People all over the world have Kundalini awakenings, and while the Fuck Zone is probably not mentioned in any Vedic texts, there are practitioners, classes, and workshops that can guide you towards having an actual Kundalini awakening if you're interested in having one. You can generate a somewhat similar effect by faking it 'til you make it. If you push yourself to expand your radar for what's sexy, you will change the radar itself to encompass all of life. One half-click to the left, and you can inhabit a brighter, more sensual universe full of sexy humans just waiting to be noticed by sexy you.

DIY: Nothing clouds your intuition and takes you out of the Fuck Zone more than being under stress. If you get stuck in 'decision gridlock,' it's a good idea to find a trusted friend to gut-check with. They will either confirm what you already know or remind you that not everything has to be decided today.

2.7: Fuck Trauma[1]

Did you have a crap-ass childhood? Welcome! Maybe you had an *okay* or even a happy childhood, but then some other horror show happened. Congrats! Maybe you've had a great life... until very recently when something went so hideously awry, and now most days feel like you're tunneling through raw sewage. Yay raw sewage! If you're not used to thinking of life's hideousness™ as a gift, as someone with a *just a dab* of trauma myself, believe me I relate. The good news is that all those nightmare life experiences, or those you wished were nightmares because then you might have woken up, may have made you more naturally intuitive.

If you grew up in alcoholism or some form of extreme chaos, you might have been rewarded with the gift of acute perception, otherwise known as intuition. As a child, if you didn't take the emotional temperature of the room, there might be danger. So you developed an ability to read people because it was your job to know

---

[1] *If you've led a charmed life and nothing bad has ever happened to you, you will still find this chapter relevant, particularly because it will help you understand others who have.*

136

what the erratic folks in your surroundings were thinking. In adulthood, you may be able to form impressions of people in a way that seems almost psychic. *When it comes to getting laid, this ability is your secret weapon.*

If your trauma happened sometime after childhood (or you're in it now) you may have seen it as an opportunity to get to the very bottom of yourself, as well as to see which people you can count on, and which you can't. This can only help you when looking at possible bed partners! You developed a more acute intuition about others, which may or may not show up to the party with its unpopular cousin, Hypervigilance (that bitch). Or even its redheaded stepchild, Paranoia (I can say that because I'm a ginger).

Some time ago there was a news story about a high school teacher who was 42 years old and left the state with his 15-year-old student, intending to have a live-in sexual relationship with her. He'd already been fired for kissing her on school premises, so I guess he figured he had nothing to lose by crossing state lines. They ran off to a hippie, polyamorous commune in California, whose inhabitants eventually reported them when they felt something was awry. You know you're being creepy when you're busted by a bunch of polyamorous nudists.

I found myself triggered by this for personal reasons. What is a trigger? It's when something shitty in the present activates something even shittier in the past. It is felt not just in the brain but also in the body (somatically) and stays in the body long after the original adrenaline-producing event is over. It's trauma that's been locked in. Many people find even the subject of sex extremely triggering. This is not a sign that there's something wrong with sex, or with them, but that the Fuck Trauma has to be moved out.

Here are some ways that are effective to shift trauma out of the body:
- EMDR
- Brainspotting
- Hypnotherapy
- Yoga
- Massage
- Rolfing with someone who understands trauma
- Somatic Experience Processing
- Talk therapy with someone who works somatically

- Intuitive healers
- Ecstatic dance
- Any form of exercise undertaken with the intention of shifting trauma

To digest triggers on a psychological level, there's a therapeutic modality called *Mentalization*, a method of 'thinking about thinking' founded by a therapist named Peter Fonagy in the 1990s, which teaches you to tease out what caused a potentially harmful emotional state. You do this by figuring out where the mental 'glitch' occurred that caused the trigger to form, then dialog rationally about it with someone who can hold space for you to process it, until you can effectively process things for yourself.

Dialectical Behavioral Therapy (DBT) developed by the brilliant Professor Marsha Linehan is another effective system to parse out the 'you' from 'what happened to you' or 'what you are currently feeling.' In 2011, Professor Linehan finally admitted that she spent decades developing her pioneering ideas to help deal with her own borderline personality tendencies. (More evidence of how having mental issues does not preclude you from being an incredible healing force in the world.)

Often people who are traumatized seek out other traumatized people. There's a heightened feeling of intensity and 'connection' that mimics some true soulmate shit but may be masking a rather vicious attachment. This is referred to as 'trauma bonding' by the patron saint of sex addiction, Dr. Patrick Carnes. I prefer the gentler definition of love coach and bestselling author Kathryn Alice, who calls this kind of mega-intense relationship "crazy love." While we all agree that this kind of dramatic entanglement is not optimal (and sometimes abusive) Kathryn believes that a shift in the relationship towards something more sustainable can be achieved if both parties are willing. Only you can decide if the sex or the love makes it worth working on the Fuck Trauma such a union can leave in its wake.

Now. If you knew a person who had at any time sexually victimized someone else, whether through rape, assault, stalking, stealthing (the practice of ripping off a condom mid-fuck) abusing, deceiving, or using someone who didn't want to be used, holding a job over someone's head unless they complied with sexual demands etc. then you would certainly make sure that person could never do that again. *So, what do you do if you suspect that person was you?*

If you know you have past sexual 'misdeeds', from relatively minor things that make you feel icky, to more serious assault or rape that has affected someone else's life permanently, make like a Catholic and find someone to confess to, if there is something to confess. **Then you must pay any price that needs to be paid.** There is no other way around this step.

You cannot move forward into getting your sexual needs met in a healthy way if you're still holding guilt that immense, or if there is that large a karmic debt to be paid. Even if you don't believe in karma, it's vital that you take the time to understand why and how those transgressions were harmful to others. You then not only vow to never commit them again, but also resolve to make your future dating life a 'living amends.' As we've seen in recent world events, denial doesn't stop the tide catching up with you eventually.

And if there's nothing to confess, *then stop acting like there is.* **Needing sex is not a crime, and you are not a criminal for wanting to get laid.** It's not necessary to develop a predator's intuition to lure someone into bed. It is not necessary to lure anyone to anything. Sleeping with someone is not a manipulative stance to acquire something or someone, or a ruse to get something that's not freely given. Don't listen to those Alpha posers; they're not on the up and up.

It's possible for someone to be a 'hunter' without being a predator. I never liked the word cougar for that reason. I know experientially that as an 'older woman' (ugh) meeting younger men was just a function of setting my Fuck Frequency to DTF.

I trust that you will use the *noticing* power for good and not for evil. Every person at some point in their lives must deal with the consequences of their own worst instincts. The day after you get laid, you still have to look at yourself in the mirror. If you see a monster looking back at you, it's probably time to change course. If you follow my guidelines, you'll know the difference. You'll feel it.

Once you've done some work to move trauma out of the body, you can choose to stay in 'I can never trust anyone again', or you could use the remaining perceptive gift to have better sex, or more of it. As much as personal triumphs can morph into Psychic Shrapnel or Torture Loops that disable us, conversely your trauma left you with a beautiful byproduct. Also, being Fuck Motivated is a powerful agent to propel us out of the self-destructive part of us that wants us to fail/be miserable/die. Use it.

Your hypervigilance can be channeled into paying close attention to what's happening to your bed partner. If you're engaging in sex with all your senses, hearing sounds, watching changes in skin color and texture, reading gestures, *you will intuitively know what to do next.* Your commitment to noticing (just like you had to in childhood) is exactly what makes you great in bed!

A new confidence can develop, knowing that your unique way of perceiving the world teaches you how to please the one you're with. And what you don't intuitively discern, you'll be motivated to find out by asking questions with the genuine curiosity and courage of the highly empathic. The *marrieds* I've coached who describe sex becoming infrequent, boring, or absent in a relationship are complaining of basically the same thing—my spouse doesn't see me, doesn't feel me, doesn't care to remember that swirly-tongue thing that got me off last time.

Isn't trauma fun? Not only are you better at figuring out your partner's (or partners') favorite proclivities, but also in communicating your own. Also, if you've processed all the shit that went down in your life, then you're not squeamish about dealing with things other people find uncomfortable. We've already been to the bottom of the shame barrel, kids— what's a bodily fluid or two?

We've already dispelled the myth that you can be too 'damaged' to find love or get laid. The truth is that your pain can scar into the beautiful gift of Sexual Intuition. If we embrace the broken parts of us, and allow those shards to glint in the sunlight, we will inevitably be more desirable because we are more true. At some point trauma might make us slutty AF, but we don't have to take that as a bad thing.

DIY: *There are books available for people with mental illness, mental health issues, or those who would like to work on starting to unpack their trauma. Here are some that I recommend, or that were recommended to me by Dr. Karol Darsa, Founder and Executive Director of Reconnect Integrative Trauma Treatment Centers:*

The Body Keeps the Score: Brain, Mind, and Body in the Healing of Trauma, by Bessel van der Kol

Waking The Tiger: Healing Trauma, by Peter A. Levine and Ann Frederick

An Unquiet Mind: A Memoir of Moods and Madness, by Kay Redfield Jamison

Codependent No More: How to Stop Controlling Others and Start Caring for Yourself, by Melanie Beattie

Women Who Hurt Themselves, by Dusty Miller

How I Stayed Alive When My Brain Was Trying to Kill Me: One Person's Guide to Suicide Prevention, by Susan Rose Blauner

Additional Resources in the U.S:
National Suicide Prevention Lifeline: *Call 1-800-273-8255*
Crisis text line: *Text TALK to 741741*
For LGBTQ: *The Trevor Project: Call 866-488-7386*
For Veterans: *Call 1-800-273-8255, Press 1*

Part 3.0: Ready, Set, Laid!

3.1: Getting Laid on the Regular

I know the title of this book suggests a level of casual fuckery, and having a *Trampage* may be exactly the palate cleanser you need or have needed at different times in your life. In this section, we will start to go into specific, intuitive actions you're going to take to get what you want. But first, without condemning hook-ups or casual sex, I'm going to suggest you expand your mindset (if you haven't already) to encompass something more committed.

Arghhhhhh.... Maybe you feel like you're not ready for a relationship, let alone marriage, children, and the slow trudge towards mortgage-driven wage slavery followed closely by death. Who could blame you? Perhaps you've been down the marriage road and a return trip sounds about as appetizing as a slice of shit pie. I get it. I've chafed against the feeling that once I commit to someone I'm no longer 'free.' However, whatever your Ideas about relationships, if you want to get laid on the reg, *the most energy-efficient way to accomplish this is in some form of relationship.*

Here are some types of relationships you may have experienced or heard of:

- FWBs: Friends with Benefits
- Fuck buddies
- Monogamous
- Consciously non-monogamous
- Monogamish (Dan Savage's term for unions that are mostly monogamous, with other allowances, such as when a heterosexual guy 'allows' his bisexual partner to date women)
- Bf/gf (Boyfriend or girlfriend)
- Partners/significant others
- Swingers
- Rotating roster of available lovers
- Polyamorous configurations like triads or pods
- Polyamorous relationships with no hierarchy when it comes to nominating 'primary partners' vs. 'secondary' or 'tertiary' partners
- 24-7 BDSM relationships such as M/s (Master/slave) or O/p (Owner/property)
- Marriage

I like to think of these monikers as describing 'structures.' The word 'relationship' conjures up confusing or negative connotations for many, for example, the way a Fuck Buddy or FWB is considered 'not a relationship' whereas a bf/gf *is* a relationship. (It's still a relationship if you're relating, isn't it?) The label is not as important as the 'structure' it represents. In fact, you can create a 'structure' with someone that works to meet both your and another person's needs and call it Cucumber, as in, "I'd like you to meet my Cucumber, Gary."

When it comes to marriage, the data may surprise you. Statistics from studies about sexual frequency and satisfaction conducted by both the Journal of Sexual Medicine and the Center for Sexual Health Promotion at Indiana University indicate married people **are having more and better sex than their single peers.** *What?* Of course, there are unique challenges as more water accumulates under the [boning] bridge, but overall it seems the marrieds are getting laid more, better, and with more variation.

It can be challenging to ask the person you brush your teeth next to if they'd like to try that cool thing you saw on World's Strangest Addictions. However, if you find someone willing to sexually explore with you from the outset this can become your joint quest, kind of like some couples collaborate on a new kitchen. Wouldn't you rather explore sexual energies than tile preferences? (Unless you want to select your tiles based on fuck durability.)

Forget what you've seen in your parents and friends that view shutting down sexually or cheating as their only two options. There's a massive smorgasbord of 'structures' limited only by your imagination. If you consciously choose to have casual sex for the rest of your life that's fine, just don't let that be the default choice because of the biggest Torture Loop of all – Fear of Commitment.

In life, when we commit to something or someone, it can provide a foundation for everything we want to achieve personally and professionally. What if you were able to find someone you *actually like* to do healthy (horizontal) dances with, based on clear boundaries around time and resources? What if a sexual relationship could actually nourish you, giving as much, or more, than it takes? If you find someone as Fuck Motivated as you are, *why not see how it goes?*

Loneliness has been proven to be a greater risk to cardiovascular health than traditionally known causes of premature death like smoking and obesity. Researchers at Brigham Young University found this increase in physical risk due to social isolation spans across ages, genders, and geographic locations. Not to be alarmist, but your idea of staying single to avoid the hassle of a relationship could wind up killing you.

There's a power in finding a compatible sexual partner, and narrowing your focus to just that person, so you can go *deeper*. (Even if you decide to add more partners to the mix, you then have an ability to go deeper with them if it's appropriate.) The self-discipline it takes to channel your sexual desires in this way means you don't have to worry about where your next fuck is coming from (keeping in mind no one owes you a fuck, even someone you're in a relationship with). Committing to 'seeing how things go,' can be a more fruitful approach than committing to running through people like they're generic multi-colored pieces of candy.

DIY: *Quiz—Do you carry any of the following widely held assumptions?*

- *There's someone out there that's 'perfect' and until I find them, it's best not to become emotionally invested in anyone.*
- *A true relationship has to be monogamous.*
- *The first sexual encounter has to be awkward.*
- *The first sexual encounter is the only exciting one.*
- *Marriages are magical places of constant happiness.*
- *Marriages cannot be happy.*
- *A Fuck Motivated woman is untrustworthy, the only woman safe to be in a relationship with is one who doesn't like sex very much.*
- *I will never find someone who likes sex as much as I do.*
- *Men can't commit because they have a 'higher sex drive.'*
- *People are expendable; there's always another person around the corner waiting to suck my (metaphorical) dick.*

Newsflash: if you believe even one of these statements is unequivocally true, you may be robbing yourself of the possibility of designing a 'structure' that works for you with someone who could actually meet your needs in the long

There's another advantage to committing to a more regular 'structure', and that is you can get tested, 'fluid-bonded' (agreeing to have unprotected sex) and settle in for some Fuck Marathons. There's no such thing as 'safe sex,' only 'safer sex,' and knowing someone better reduces that day-after 'throw the dice' feeling of multiple anonymous hook-ups.

It's important to add that STIs are like colds and flus, but because they manifest on the genitals we're taught to think of them as shameful. In fact, they're like any recurring health condition to manage and treat, as long as you don't bury them in denial. You're obligated to disclose to a potential partner but your STI panel doesn't reflect anything about your 'purity' or 'cleanliness,' nor is it a judgment on how many partners you've had, or haven't had.

DIY: *When researching your or a partner's STI, be careful with whom you trust as your sources. You may have already noticed that the internet is not a reliable diagnostic tool, so make sure you're tested by a doctor or at a health center. Approach with caution any info you see online after a diagnosis. Not only is* *some information given with a shaming or sex-negative bend, but even 'reputable' sources may be sticking with a highly conservative agenda. STIs are extremely common, very treatable, and may even be an opportunity to reach new levels of empathy and communication. The reality is if you discount people with herpes or HPV to have a relationship with, your choices may be limited to almost no one between the ages of 15 and 49.*

Many dating coaches or love experts approach sex as if it were a dirty afterthought, or worse, some kind of bargaining chip. I've coached and spoken with countless married people that walked down the aisle with an unconscious knowing (but refusal to admit) the warning signs of sexual incompatibility that would eventually become relationship deal breakers. You don't have to be one of them, not least because it's very difficult to get a refund for wedding cake.

Once you attract someone who has a matching Fuck Frequency, don't just bail if the sex is hot but you have 20 Ideas about why a relationship with them won't work, instead try exploring your mutual Fuck Energies *with heart*. Dare to go outside your comfort zone and you might be rewarded with someone who will expend some effort to make time to get you off, as well as a new kind of 'comfort zone' in the increasingly stressful and isolating world many of us inhabit.

Advertisers present us with an aspirational 'vanilla' world with a white dress, babies, and a Dodge Caravan in the driveway, but if you're like me, your idea of heaven is much pervier. A great relationship *can* be based on mutual Fuck Motivation, because for some people shared interests, values, intellectual compatibility, and even a terrific mileage SUV are not enough.

A Fuck Motivated person, aka slut, will suck your actual/metaphorical/psychic dick like no other, because said slut is smart, already likes you, and will work hard to figure out what you like. If you find a good slut, and are one yourself, why not use how much you both enjoy fucking as the impetus to explore a more ongoing situation? I'm not saying LTRs are the only valid life choice, just urging you to tune into your intuition enough to hear a voice that whispers, "Stay..."

There's nothing wrong with relying on *Limerance*, the fluffy, golden infatuation period that poly people call *NRE* (New Relationship Energy) as the ultimate turn-on. But for many other folks, the fucking improves as the intimacy deepens. Love ain't all that bad! I almost called this book 'How to Get Laid or Get Love Using Your Intuition' but didn't because I *intuited* that if I did, some of you might not be here with me right now. The point is, be open to your intuition guiding you to *both*...

3.2: There's Someone Thinking About Fucking You RN

Unless you grew up trapped in a basement (and if you did, I'm sorry!) it's likely that at this very moment, there's a special *someone* obsessing over why they didn't get to fuck you in high school. Maybe they're replaying that stolen thing that you did in middle school with a different ending than the gym teacher catching you (in the fantasy, she joined in!). This *someone* may not match up with your idea of who you should be with but is nevertheless willing and able to do some kind of dirty with you. Your intuition can help you find them, as well as letting them find you.

When we have a concrete idea of what the person we date should look like, instead of focusing on what they *feel* like, we miss a lot. Everyone falls into the idea trap at some point, even people who married their college sweethearts. At some point we form an attachment to a *concept* of something, as opposed to a person. The worst part about that is that the sex suffers, and that's because you can't actually fuck a concept (God knows I've tried).

Most people are inauthentic about what drives them. Being inauthentic happens all the time in relationships, either to avoid hurting someone's feelings, or to avoid scaring ourselves. We develop workarounds for our limiting beliefs like choosing porn over people, money over sexual chemistry, or pragmatism over passion. We lie.

One of my clients, Chloe, is a brilliant and beautiful woman in her 40's who is divorced with two young children. Her ex-husband is a CEO type, in this case you can follow the bouncing ball along the character traits: narcissist, ambitious, driven, distracted, someone who had to be 'handled.' In her post-divorce dating life, this cool blonde with a high IQ tended to lust after the same kind of man. She gravitated towards the high flyers/rollers and egomaniacs, and while she had some fun experiences (especially with much younger men) she was starting to feel 'crispy.'

After being burned (to a crisp) by yet another commitment-phobe that took her down a rabbit hole of kink without being responsible for her aftercare, Chloe was surprised to hear from Chris, an old classmate that had apparently been lusting after her for decades. Cautiously, they began talking on the phone, and found themselves up until all hours with much to share. This man did not fit the profile of what my client imagined for herself (he cobbled together a living from many jobs and was by no means wealthy) but I urged her to be patient and stay open.

When Chris drove from another state to take her to a concert, she knew he was serious. Over time he also showed himself to be seriously interested in exploring kink with her, as well as taking on a supportive, nurturing role with her children, freeing her up to be Oprah to his Steadman. Chris and Chloe are currently in a fabulous, loving relationship, where I can report, one nocturnal fuck session recently broke some of the cabinet hinges in her kitchen. (I didn't ask how exactly, I'm just glad she's happy.)

If you want to invite passion into your life it might just entail having a deep personal shift. If you're a *Cerebral*, forget finding something or someone that looks 'good on paper.' You might learn to soften, without having to become soft. If you're more of an *Emotional*, you get to keep your feelings, and also express all parts of yourself when it comes to sex (some people are aroused by crying, so it's all good). If you're a *Genital*, stop pathologizing your desires, categorizing your urges as 'addiction' or 'excess.' Why do you have to diagnose yourself? **Maybe you're just horny.**

Only you can give yourself permission to experience radically awesome fucking with someone who could also have a partnership with you. A state of being that is always **allowing** and **noticing**, as opposed to **denying** and **justifying**, invites the kind of people you may have overlooked before, whose needs might dovetail into your own. Writing out her needs is the exercise I had Chloe do before she found Chris, and in this way she began to understand that her basic need for 'Security' could be met emotionally in ways that didn't have to include timeshare in a private jet.

In my decades living in America it's hard to miss the work ethic we espouse that promotes a certain type of effort, leading to an expected trajectory of progress and reward. The whole Puritan ideal is damaging in more ways than just convincing us there's something wrong with wanting sex, it makes us think we're guaranteed a certain outcome if we work hard enough. (This is also known as entitlement.)

Intuitive work does not necessarily involve 'doing,' it is also *ontological* (i.e. a change in 'being'). This ontological shift can be more effective than running around desperately trying to make things happen. Sometimes it's as simple as realizing when someone is attracted to you. Many people have no idea when a friend or co-worker desires them. At this very moment, there may be someone waving you in for take-off with orange flags on the runway, only you're too busy staring at the pretty lights.

There are also those who think *everyone* is attracted to them or that *no one ever* is. Once again, be on the lookout for absolutes in your thinking, as they are *never* true. (Okay, rarely.)

Conversely, it's important you stop painfully 'waiting out' certain friendships to see if they'll turn into sex. I promise if you're supposed to get laid with someone in your life, it will be clear, intuitive, and natural. There's a deliberate vagueness we indulge in when it comes to people we're attracted to, instead of being direct and finding out what the deal is, because we believe that the truth is worse. The greatest gift someone can give you when it's apparent there's no shot with them, is to allow you to use that bandwidth for somebody else. Just don't be surprised if it's someone you already have a past with, who also wants some kind of future.

DIY: *When you are listening for an intuitive hit, the important thing is not to question it. Again 'first thought, best thought'—you can't move forward from that first thought if you waste time questioning it. Did someone specific occur to you when reading this chapter? You may choose to reconnect with them* (without attachment) *to see if a flame can be re-kindled or continues to exist between you. Why not? We're all going to shuffle off this planet any second, so go big because we're all going 'home' anyway.*

3.3: Online Shenanigans

Online dating is no more 'unnatural' than meeting someone IRL, but sending out a missive to a potential bedmate can still be a massive mindfuck. Even responding once someone has swiped you (signaling they may find you moderately to severely attractive) requires more finesse than most of us are born with. At least one third of relationships in the US now start online, so you got this! If you've been practicing the exercise at the end of the Fuck Energy chapter, you might find yourself mastering 'reading between the lines' when checking out a pic or profile. There's no need to suffer or overthink it, and these simple guidelines should set you on your way...

◆ **No dick pics, please:** For most of us the dick is not a disembodied piece of meat. The reason we like *your* dick is because it's yours, and maybe that's the reason you like it too. (Or don't like it.) When we're attracted to you, we would maybe love see your cock, but *even then* we may still never want a picture of it. If we do fancy a pic, it's only when we're good and ready. We need to get mentally prepared. If we're older we might need time to put our reading glasses on. (If we're really old, it might be a monocle.)

If you have a dick and that's solely what someone is interested in you for, they might ask to *inspect* it, but that's a whole other energy—from someone who wishes to be serviced and will let you know that up front. Sometimes I think the kind of men who send unsolicited dick pics harbor an unconscious desire for either humiliation or to Dominate with their sexuality. If you want to force people to do stuff (or be forced) you would be better served to hang out in BDSM clubs or join communities on Fetlife with people who share those perfectly valid kinks. (Keep in mind a kink-friendly location or website is *still* not implied consent for unveiling a penis bomb).

If we don't know you, or we *do* know you but aren't attracted to you, or even if we think you're hot shit, it's perfectly valid for us not to be *forced* to see your dick-piece, even if it's **astounding** in your opinion. Not sure what percentage of women men estimate will see a dick and uncontrollably throw their hand/mouth/vagina at it, but whatever the estimate, it's *high*. If you're a man who sends other men you want to bang dick pics they didn't ask for, that's also a consent violation. If you send someone a picture of your pussy, that's just marketing. (I'm kidding, everyone relax, of course the same goes for a non-consensual vulva.)

+ **Be genuine:** One of the things that really chaps my ass is the way certain 'experts' claim to have the last word on how to create 'the perfect profile' on a dating app. These are often based on what 'all women' or 'all men' respond to or find attractive. While I myself help people with dating profiles in a coaching capacity, the only 'perfect profile' is one that expresses you perfectly.

If you're going to use a picture from five years ago, then say it's a picture from five years ago. If you've put on a few pounds, or gotten older, get new pictures taken that reflect that (professional ones if you're not a great selfie-taker). The idea is not to 'trick' someone into meeting with you with a false carrot, nor is working off some listicle that told you '3 Top Mistakes Women Make With Men with Manbuns' or '7 Things Men Look For in a Chicken Baster.' The sooner you let go of the retrograde gender tropes, the sooner you can become curious about how you're going to connect with the actual person in front of you. Your intuition can take in a lot about how traditional or progressive a person is *sometimes within seconds of meeting them*, and the last thing you want to do is 'pretend accordingly.'

+ **Be specific:** Don't just spew fawning, sickly garbage at someone because it's what you think they want to hear. (I would be shocked if any online greeting that started with, "Hi Dear" ever got anyone laid, unless the sender's magnetism is so astounding that they're already dodging panty throwers in the street.) A good rule is if you know nothing about the person you're approaching, *don't approach* until you have a general sense of who they are, by looking at their profile properly and letting your intuition guide you. Use their name, not 'dear,' 'lovely,' or 'beautiful.' Generalities don't work because everyone knows a 'lazy looker is also a lazy licker.' (Don't look for that one on InspirationQuotes.org, I made it up.)

I get more than my share of approaches from strangers (including unsolicited dick pics) even though I'm 43 years old and my Facebook status clearly states I'm in a relationship. Here's an odd missive I got recently on FB Messenger from someone I've never met:

Hello. I had gone thru your profile and it seems like you have a good head on your shoulders i [sic] would love to learn more about you my name is [redacted]

Okay [redacted] I get it—you're desperate and horny and don't view grammar as a priority. You sent 500 of these messages indiscriminately because you're convinced women are thinking, "If only there was a man who could see how *sensible* I am, where, where oh where is he?"

In comedy the number one rule is to be able to *read the room*. Same goes for the internet. Know your medium. It's Facebook, not a dating app, but it's possible Svetlana from Latvia has been waiting for [redacted] her whole life to transport both herself and her teenage son Dragomir to the US of A. (If acquiring a bride from another country is something you see for yourself—maybe even out of a basic Need to Rescue/Be Rescued—I've known a few happy marriages that started this way. Again, not a service Facebook offers. Find an agency, or wanted ads, or just book a plane ticket and go get that Belarusian Barbie/Georgian GI Joe of your dreams!)

No matter what connection you think you have with a person, if you haven't actually met them, that connection is, for now, just in your head. They don't feel it. They don't know you. *They're not in the story yet.*

♦ **Don't kiss ass:** No-one wants insincere flattery, especially that which seeks to elevate us into the realm of a deity. Unless deities can get laid too, this is not useful. Here's an example of an actual message on Facebook that doesn't work:

Greetings Susanna! I am in awe of your celestial wonderment. God blessed you in making you more beautiful than an ambiance of dreams. May all that you have envisioned for yourself become a reality, Amen. Be blessed and smile!
[Name redacted, but it didn't matter because he was banned from FB the following week, I'm guessing for a message that was less 'celestial.']

He gets points for using my name, and even spelling it right. After that, zero points, negative points, if I had balls they would have retracted into my anus amount of points. He even added that age-old ultimate clit-boner killer urging me to *smile*.

No one wants to be sprayed with Flattery Shrapnel like some kind of indiscriminate compliment sprinkler. If you really like someone, take the time to tell 'em what it is you appreciate (this works in a relationship too). Remark on the stuff about them *they* haven't even considered loving, stuff that lets them know you're receptive to their Fuck Frequency like, "I'm digging how that birthmark on your neck is shaped like the former Soviet Union."

People don't want to be approached by phony reverence because it doesn't bode well for getting their actual needs met. Even when it's real reverence, who the fuck could keep up with an image of perfection? The minute a fart escaped, it would be *over*. All of us want to feel we can relax with someone, not walk around with an ambiance of celestial whatever the fuck. Also, this kind of ass-kissing makes us think we're being trolled or catfished, which we probably are.

So, how do you make someone want to know you? You can't, in the sense that you can't *make* anyone do anything. However, if you state your case in an authentic way that says you're actually *taking in* what a person is about; *seeing*, *noticing* and *receiving* them in a way that feels **specific**, you're more likely to have a shot. Not many people want to be treated as just than someone's object or fucktoy. Of course, some people *only* want to be fucktoys, but that's a very specific fetish and there's no way to know they want that with you, even if their Instagram features 170 close-ups of their ass.

◆ **Offer something real:** Once you introduce yourself, lead with what works best about you, and be honest about what you're interested in. Offer something of yourself and be prepared to share what you're really about. Do you wear cravats? Smoke a pipe? Take acid? Disclose this, but you don't have to lead with the acid unless their profile pic is trippy. How much specific stuff can you notice about the person? Are they into R.Crumb? Croquet? Maggot play? Just take a moment without *stalking* someone to form an impression of this human being. And then don't **expect** anything.

Practice reaching out to people you'd like to get to know on Facebook, Instagram, or whatever other digital platform has sprung up since I started writing this sentence. Do it *without* a romantic endgame in mind, maybe just something that says you appreciate their energy. Preferably you have mutual friends, already follow each other, or have met, but please don't just message them with "Hi" or "Hey." "Hi" is not sufficient; it's like throwing a 20-pound barbell at someone they didn't ask for, then wondering why they aren't grateful for only one black eye.

You have to *spot* a person, conversationally speaking, like you would a bench-pressing bud. Send an honest paragraph ONCE, and be prepared for no response. If you get a reply, be ready to do the heavy lifting and have an actual conversation. Your crush is not a thing, a collection of abs, or a pair of tits with eyes. This is a human who may well want to get laid, not unlike yourself. Worst-case scenario, if you approach with respect, you might make a friend. And you know how friends love setting their friends up with other nice friends...

You have nothing to lose if you reach out and the person isn't interested in cravats and pipes, but if you reach out with enthusiasm and sincerity, I happen to know of at least three happy monogamous couples, and some polyamorous folks for whom Facebook worked/works perfectly for meeting likeminded Facefuckers.

- **Make someone feel safe:** We've already covered the importance of safety as a basic need for many. When it comes to dating or hook-up apps, be aware that for those of us who identify as women (especially trans women), any time we don't get chopped up in pieces and incinerated after meeting someone off the internet, it's a *win*! Keeping this in mind, *do* convey a sense of physical safety, and even better, that you're in touch with objective reality. Someone needs to know she's safe to be in public or private with you. If you can't manage to get that across in an early convo, it's probably going to be a non-starter, especially on hook-up apps like Tinder.

Keep in mind that men can also be turned off if someone makes them feel emotionally unsafe, such as by signs that if things don't go as planned, it will bring down Armageddon. Always ask yourself, "Would I do/say/behave like this IRL?" and "Am I expecting too much from this person?" Some people think they can get away with all kinds of fuckery when hiding behind a keyboard. (Not many guys would actually flash their peen to a woman first thing on a first date, although it seems like we may have underestimated that one as well...)

People smell inauthenticity like too much cologne unless they're wearing too much perfume to notice. Dousing yourself energetically with something strong or fake is inevitably trying to mask something else, something you don't have to be afraid to present because it's uniquely and unmistakably you. But when you do get a date, make time for a shower. You don't have to be that authentic.

DIY : Guess what? You can harness your Sexual Intuition when looking at pictures on a dating app. This is something people pay me to do, but I got good at it through practice, so I know you can too. Just allow yourself to sense what is beyond the images and words presented. Pay attention to facts, such as someone avoiding looking at the camera in every shot, the locations they choose, and what they're trying to convey by choosing those particular images to share. It's important to give yourself as much context as you can when looking for intuitive hits, as you're not trying to be psychic. When you meet up with people, and as you get to know them, it's a great opportunity to check in verbally to validate how many of your intuitive 'hits' about them were correct. So the person you were sure was perfect for you didn't message you back, or worse, ended up just Photoshopping his head on the body of a snake handler—don't be discouraged! It just means you're closer to the next right hunch and your next great fuck, from a true reptile owner, not some phony.

3.4: What Are You Available For?

Getting laid requires a willingness to be intimate, both with yourself and someone else. Just the act of taking (some of) your clothes off in front of a potential bedmate might require uncharacteristic boldness. If you're mature enough to be (even partially) naked with someone, you must be naked enough to ask them, ***"What are you available for?"***

Then watch. Not only watch, but also *observe intuitively*, without judging *what it all means.* Don't take something someone says and run with it. An example of this is taking the fact that a person has never been married or married five times as evidence to form a die-hard opinion about their character. Whatever thing you've been led to believe about 'girls with cats' or 'dudes who ride hoverboards' has not been substantiated about this particular human yet, though they can certainly factor into a hunch.

You may choose to intersperse *"What are you available for?"* with other salient questions like:
- What's your name?
- What generation are you?
- What are you into?

- When was the last time you were tested?
- How did your last relationship end?
- Have you ever had a relationship?
- Been married?
- Got kids?
- Want kids?
- Are you a kid? (As in, literally, under 18?)
- How was your last sexual experience?
- Are you into monogamy/misogyny/Merlot?
- Are you lying to someone by being here?
- Are you happy?
- What is the weirdest thing you wouldn't want me to know about you?

Of course, if you don't want to know any of these things, it's perfectly okay (other than the safe/old enough to have sex part.) Also, you probably don't want to fire off all these questions at once, or just use them as a guideline for checking out their social media. (This isn't stalking, it's reconnaissance.)

Pay attention, for sooner rather than later, people will reveal exactly what they're down for, simply by what they can sustain. The amount of bandwidth they have will be obvious

SO shortly, if you can just keep it in your pants a little while longer... Whether you want a 'casual' encounter or something more, there's no substitute for consciously and methodically getting to know someone a little bit, before you release the hounds of oxytocin and everything goes to holy heaven/hell. (As always, confirm your 'intuitive hits' with whatever words and actions ensure your own safety.)

DIY: *Now that you're preparing to pose that question to someone else, here is the ultimate ball-kicker, so you might like to settle in with a hot beverage and a notebook to dig in. I'll wait... Okay now* **pose that very question to yourself.** *What am I REALLY available for? (Add that REALLY, just to make sure you're paying attention):*

1. *Do I want some version of getting laid on the reg?*
2. *What kind of time and bandwidth do I have?*
3. *What kind of sex turns me on?*
4. *What gender roles or sexualities do I currently enjoy, or wish I could explore?*
5. *Is there anything else I need to know about myself, and how I behave in dating situations?*

Don't try to fake yourself out with flowery pronouncements and grand ideas of what you SHOULD want because of what you think is possible for you. What needs are you trying to meet? Who are you going to have to be to get those needs met? What makes you happy? When you frame your new self-awareness about your preferences, always ask "What?" but never "Why?" Why? Because it doesn't matter why you find a gap between the two front teeth sexy, just that you do. (It's called a diastema FYI.) The point is you're your own life partner, the only one who will most certainly be there at the end, so you need to know these things.

You can get great intuitive hits from messaging with someone (especially as you tune up your instrument with practice) but keep in mind that until you actually meet in person, it's all academic. If you can't meet in person, because they live in another country, city or town, you may want to check in via Skype, Facetime, or some other videocall platform, so you're not just analyzing someone's emojis. Once you hear a tone of voice or observe body language, it becomes easier to sense clues about how genuine they're being with all those 'heart eyes.' Ideally, once you meet or voice-call, you can refer back to their already stated 'deal,' to let your gut confirm if it really *is* their deal, or they're just addicted to that purple devil with the horns.

Don't just take mental notes, but *energetic* ones. (This might seem like it's not specific, but hopefully your Fuck Energy senses have learned how to tingle and you know exactly what I'm talking about.) Witness the behavior, not just the words, the breath and the pupils dilating (they do that with desire, see?). Really undertake a scientific exploration of What This Person Can Share With You At This Time. You may not want anything more than forty-five minutes with them, but it's *still* advisable to know what they're up for.

Now, TRUST. You're not a mind reader, and being able to listen to your intuition doesn't promise that (although it can lead to an almost psychic sense of awareness.) Your intuition can guide you towards not only to how exactly this exchange is going to get everyone's needs met, but also to whether someone's a narcissistic master manipulator. By feeling into this *before* you sleep with them, you can be realistic about where someone might fit (ha) even if you already know they're not going to part of any future life plans.

You want to get *specific* about:

- Whether this person wants a relationship.
- Whether if you fuck them, you're also sleeping over, or they are.
- What kind of time they have available for getting laid, and how much of it they might be willing to spend with you.
- What kind of sex they prefer.
- What genders they tend to date.
- Anything else they choose to disclose that can give you a better idea of what you're getting into if you fuck them.

Gone are the days when unstated intentions and vagueness were considered sexy. Honesty and clarity are the antidote for the disturbing epidemic of people not even realizing *in hindsight* that they didn't have someone's enthusiastic consent. We need to be responsible for ourselves, and with others, though of course charm, flirtation, and unstated dirty thoughts are just fine. Enthusiastic consent does not 'ruin the mood,' it *is* the mood. Being direct is how we get agency over our own perversions, so those same perversions don't end up owning us.

DIY: You can also use intuition to check-in and ask **yourself** if a potential partner seems to be:

- Sexually compatible with you as far as you can feel in your body, and from other questions you may have asked such as, "Do you like _____?" "What kind of touch do you like?" "What are you looking for?" "Are you kinky?"
- Someone who is capable of a relationship.
- Someone who has no interest in or capability for a relationship right now but can manage a one-off encounter.
- Available once a week/every two weeks to have sex (more about this in the last chapter.)

3.5: The Next Right Action is an Action

Perhaps you think of getting laid as a 'male' expression, but my female friends and I have been using it since we were teenagers, because chicks need to get laid too *obvi*. The idiom 'getting laid' derives from Madams Ada and Minna Everleigh, Victorian sisters whose names were co-opted for their eponymous high-end Chicago brothel. If you want to get Everleigh-ed, one magical key is to take actions with the complete belief in an eventual positive outcome.

Sometimes we get hung up on whether the thing we *think* we should do next is the *right* thing. I want to give you another way of looking at what you're doing today, by seeing it in the context of, "Is this getting me closer, or further away from getting my needs met?" Regardless of what happens, it's always a win when you choose to behave like who you want to be along the way.

Your projection of future reality influences the way you feel, speak, and behave, and therefore the results you manifest in the present. This assumption is used in everything from Neuro-linguistic Programming (NLP), to

12-Step-Programs, to the Pentecostal church. It's even used by that one nice kid on the YouTube. If you believe in a positive outcome, your next action will be intuitive- instead of fear-based, and therefore it's *always* the next right action.

Working backwards from a pessimistic belief stops you, not only because it's depressing AF, but also because it keeps you from *doing stuff*. You need to *do stuff* to have the pleasure of other people, because sadly you can't order a person from home the way you order Thai food (though you can certainly swipe left and entice them with your extremely comfy couch.) Also, taking the emotional risk of being honest and vulnerable actually qualifies as 'doing stuff.'

Everything you do can be geared towards the objective of becoming the kind of person that knows how to show up for someone, both physically and emotionally. This requires more than good intentions (or dirty ones). That's why I have always said I don't believe in the idea of 'casual sex.' All sex has some level of intimacy to it, even if sometimes that means paying attention to when another person needs to be fucked without intimacy. *Capiche?*

The person who first coined the phrase, "What would you do if you knew you could not fail?" was the Christian minister Robert H. Schuller with the popular Sunday morning TV show 'Hour of Power.' While he probably didn't anticipate it being used for perverted purposes, you can be what Killer Mike raps on the immortal Run The Jewels 3, "... a *pervert with purpose* that makes you question your purpose."

If you were working towards an ultimate destination of 'the perfect sexperience' (whatever that is to you) what would your actions look like today? How about a week from Thursday? Do they match up with what you want to create, or are you kinda full of it? Can you put aside whatever pressures you're feeling in your life to go after something better? (Yes you can, even if it's not today, most definitely a week from Thursday.)

At the end of this chapter, you might take the time to write down what you would be doing today, this week, this month, and this year, as if the future reality of "I'm going to get laid" were assured. *This is not the same as thinking you're entitled to some kind of result.* Regardless of the outcome of each one of those micro-actions, even if some of them fail spectacularly, you are still on course if you're moving. You don't have control over the results (especially when it comes to another's consent). You're just letting a positive future motivate you in the present. Here are some examples to get you started...

10 Proactive Things You Can Do Today to Increase Your Probability of Getting Laid Tomorrow:

1. **Know Thyself.** Complete this sentence "I am available for_____, and open to _____, though I definitely am not down for _____."

2. **Know what you're looking for.** Write about your ideal sexual relationship or encounter, using as much detail as possible. Don't censor yourself, just write. Engage in an honest inquiry into what you find appealing in people, both sexually and otherwise, by focusing on how someone **carries themselves**, as opposed to just physical traits.

3. **Educate yourself.** About the human body. About specific ways you could

please someone from a biological standpoint. About different lifestyle choices and how they interact with consent. If you can get online you have access to thousands of years of information, as well as the most current. Some books you may want to read are *She Comes First: The Thinking Man's Guide to Pleasuring a Woman* by Ian Kerner, *The Ultimate Guide To Anal Sex For Women* and *Opening Up* both by Tristan Taormino, and *Mating in Captivity* by Esther Perel. Keep in mind, that while many people claim to have the 'answers' about the appropriate biological 'tips' for a certain gender, your intuition can always guide you to cherry pick which of these apply to the specific person you find yourself with. You can also try O.School, an online sex education platform that is free or pay what you can, and committed to giving folks the sex education they never got.

4. **Take care of your health.** You might have some physical impediments to having sex such as erectile dysfunction, menopausal dryness, incontinence on orgasm, or any combination of these. If

so, it's a good idea to rule out physical causes before looking into underlying energetic or emotional issues. If you're a penis owner and you cum a lot, take zinc. If you're a vulva haver, slam the probiotics to protect your vag flora. Get used to seeing your genitals and reproductive system as an essential part of you that needs attention and care, as opposed to the vaguely scary 'down there.'

5. **Take care of your appearance with love.** Even in the less superficial places in the world, it's always a good move to think about the sights, sounds, and smells another person will encounter when they fuck you. You can groom and deal with whatever foliage seems errant to you, but remember that whatever set-up you go for, it's because that's what makes YOU feel sexy. There are plenty of people that fancy a natural bush, other untamed hirsuteness, or exactly what you're rocking. Rather than trying to anticipate some subjective beauty standard, take care of yourself because you're worth taking care of. The answer

to the question, "Would you want to fuck you?" should be a resounding, "Yes!"

6. **Make peace with any areas of yourself you find unseemly.** I recommend reading *Curvy Girl's Guide to Sex* by Elle Chase for everyone; it will change your perception of what we're fed by the media as 'hot,' especially if you're in a larger body and need to work on loving/accepting that. I dated someone a long time ago who used to say, "It's just tissue" and he was so much fun in bed because of his laid-back attitude to all those messy fluids flying around—*just tissue*.

7. **Get out of your apartment.** Yes, your couch is lovely, and your Netflix cue beckons, but you must at some point leave your domicile to attract what you say you want (see: Fuck Motivated). Once you know the kind of person you want to meet for sex/dating/fisting, join groups where people like that may congregate. You can be optimistic that you and your dream lover will '*meet-cute*' (a romantic first meeting scenario seen in a romcom, like ice-skating into

someone in Central Park) but you can make that more likely by narrowing down what kind of person you'd like to meet cutely. Join groups without being the kind of asshole who's just there trying to 'pick-up.' Examples include knitting circles, cuddle parties, sex-positive groups, churches, religious temples, meet-ups, hobby-related clubs, BDSM clubs, sex clubs... (I guess those are hobbies).

8. **Know what you offer**. Another one to curl up with a notebook for... List your own good qualities, both in bed and out of it, and remind yourself often. It's helpful to have an accurate picture of what delightfulness you bring, even for a night. Part of owning your shit is owning the good stuff.

9. **Lead with what you're good at.** Write down the nice things people have said to you, regarding sex or otherwise, and keep a running list. Rather than thinking of a date or the early stages of a relationship as the time to be 'on your best behavior,' think of it as wowing someone with the hors d'oeuvres (*whore*

d'oeuvres?) to whet their appetite for the main course. This is one of the reasons I don't believe in prescribed waiting periods to have sex, because Sexual Intuition will guide you to the right time on a case-by-case basis. If your specialty is giving head, then by all means unveil it early. (If you're paying attention you won't assume that 'most people like to get head' is implied consent, but find creative ways to ask such as, "Can I lick your pussy now?")

10. **Give online dating another chance.** Okay, there's this thing called the internet and it can be rather a great way to meet people. Remember that what you perceive as rejection might just be someone not answering because they're already in a monogamous relationship and just haven't de-activated their account yet, among a million other possible explanations, *none of which have anything to do with your self-worth*. You can research which apps work best for what purpose (Christian Farmer Mingle) and don't forget Facebook (with the caveats in the Online Shenanigans chapter).

Dr. Dan Siegel, a clinical psychiatry professor with whom I was privileged enough to study Mindfulness Awareness at UCLA coins the term "the neurons that fire together, wire together" to explain how a pattern of having the same thoughts influences your brain's structure over time. The good news is by taking different actions in the present, you are *literally changing your brain chemistry* to become someone who is worthy, willing, and wired to 'get lucky.' It turns out getting lucky doesn't have much to do with luck at all...

DIY: *Now go ahead and write out your positive actions, using my examples if you'd like, but always working backwards from the future reality where you're getting your Needs met. Before you know it, that future reality will be NOW. This exercise is not about pushing you into overwhelm about yet another to do list, it's a gentle nudge to your intuition that you're willing to point your compass towards wherever it wants you to go.*

Actions to Take Today With Certainty:

1.

2.

3.

4.

5.

6.

7.

8.

9.

10.

Longer Term Actions:

1.

2.

3.

4.

5.

6.

7.

8.

9.

10.

Chapter 3.6: Ambivalence

Ambivalence means being in two minds, sometimes literally feeling two opposing feelings about someone or something. Ambivalence is also a great protection for not getting your feelings hurt, and can be an excuse for not taking action. In terms of your sex, dating, and love relationships, Ambivalence is like cancer.

Ambivalence is a virus that attaches itself to whatever person you're either considering being with or already with. In this way it's similar to anger; when someone has an angry personality, it's always present, just waiting for someone else to inflame it. Ambivalence comes from a primitive coping strategy that keeps you separate from people instead of connecting with them.

Ambivalence is the reason why we can get hooked on 'avoidant' types of people over and over, because at least we're *choosing* to get rejected, the way a student who doesn't study so can tell herself she would have aced the test if she'd tried. If you feel like you're chasing someone who is slower to warm to you, you may find that even once they do show a higher level of interest, Ambivalence shows up.

Attraction is not psychological, it's energetic. There's no point analyzing why you're attracted to John but not Ringo, but if you have a recurring pattern that disappoints you over and over again it's worth taking some time to figure that shit out. It's not just that you "like bad boys" or "have a thing for cool blondes" you might be deliberately choosing people you know aren't DTF so you don't have to risk getting close to them. (Bonus: you get to be right about Torture Loop 52A "I'm a piece of shit..." or 52B "It's never gonna happen...")

In dating, Ambivalence can take the form of being excessively picky or critical about people. We pick out one small thing about someone and use that to discount the possibilities with them, "I didn't like the way she chewed her linguini," "He had this hairy mole on his arm," or "God, I cannot with the Members Only jacket." All of these things are fine to think, share with friends, and even remark on with humor, as long as you don't think they represent he complete picture.

It's perfectly valid if you dig in and notice you don't have matching Fuck Energy with someone, and decide *in your body* that you don't want to do sexy things with them. Just keep in mind that if everyone you meet is filtered through the sunglasses of Ambivalence, then no one will be good enough, attractive enough, or special enough for you. (Conversely, why would someone this great want to date someone as flawed as you?)

If you're reading this like, "I just want to get my rocks off, lady, I don't care who it is," I'm surprised you're still reading! I'm asking you to reflect on the possibility that you've had crushes on unattainable people precisely *because they were unattainable.* You picked them, *knowing* you couldn't *have* them. The attraction you feel for them is really for something missing in yourself, so even if they turned around and became completely available, you wouldn't gain the precious thing you're looking for.

A sign of emotional maturity is being able to hold two opposing thoughts at the same time. Like, "I want to be in a relationship" but also, "I don't want to be in a relationship." This is a mature and considered response, because relationships are a lot of work. Where we struggle is when the two opposing thoughts stop us from getting laid, because every person and every experience has to attain some kind of perfection.

I have a friend, Louise, who's been married for more than a decade and struggles with almost continual Ambivalence about her husband. They have a great sexual relationship, but she struggles with a recurring obsession with young dudes. When her husband agreed to an open relationship for a time, Louise got involved with avatars of 'hot guys' who demolished her emotionally because they were so unavailable. In the interests of the marriage and her own mental health, Louise and her husband decided to close the marriage, but what remained was her constant questioning of why her husband had to be older, smoke pot, be overweight, and and and...

This woman is married to the perfect partner for her, and she's achieving great things in her career as a visual artist. This isn't a question of not following her instincts, everything about their lives together works incredibly well;

they're best friends, have a great sex life, and are mutually supportive, yet she suffers. A lot.

Louise's husband has an at times debilitating immune illness, rendering him unable to walk a block on certain days. She takes this completely in her stride—without drama or self-pity—even though sometimes she has to take care of him physically. She also expresses no emotion about his condition (and she is an Emotional) rationally finding new Western and alternative ways that might help him.

One day, I mentioned to Louise that instead of dealing with her terror about her husband becoming ill and dying, she puts that energy into feeling Ambivalent about him. It is her protection, and also her hell. Once she was able to process some of the feelings underneath—pain, sadness, panic—it eased her guilt about picking apart her husband in her mind. The more she was able to *be with* the thoughts, the more she detached from them, while continuing to explore her obsession with young men (and their cocks) in her art.

Your Sexual Intuition is not Ambivalent, it knows exactly what it wants. Your Sexual Intuition clearly propels you towards someone or something. You will feel it *in your bones*. It's only your 'rational' brain holding you back when something seems outlandish or fucked up. Every relationship and many hook-ups start with something bizarre, or at the very least in a way you didn't expect. Being wholeheartedly open to whatever arises creates the 'absolute certainty' that is the antidote to ambivalence.

Question your Ambivalence if it holds you back from getting your needs met. See it as another Torture Loop, or Psychic Shrapnel, something you notice, but don't engage with too much. If you're 'not sure' you're attracted to someone, or 'not sure' if they're good for you, consider that your Sexual Intuition already knows the answer, you're just ignoring it because it seems safer than putting your shoulder behind your intention fully.

So how do you cure Recurring Ambivalence Syndrome? See how easy it is to come up with diagnoses? Just don't Google it looking for a pill to take—'Certainta cures your doubts, ask your doctor.' A better cure is to keep noticing. What we struggle against gives it power, what we ignore leads to delusion. Just the awareness of what you do will lead to a change in your Fuck Frequency. Institute a generous, but somewhat neutral observer within you, and (as any hypnotherapist will tell you) eventually your subconscious mind will get bored with the same old pattern and choose something (or someone) different.

I often think about the quote by singer and author Portia Nelson:

"I walk down the street.
There is a deep hole in the sidewalk.
I fall in.
I am lost... I am helpless.
It isn't my fault.
It takes forever to find a way out.

I walk down the same street.
There is a deep hole in the sidewalk.
I pretend I don't see it.
I fall in again.
I can't believe I am in the same place.
But, it isn't my fault.
It still takes me a long time to get out.

I walk down the same street.
There is a deep hole in the sidewalk.
I see it is there.
I still fall in. It's a habit.
My eyes are open.

I know where I am.
It is my fault. I get out immediately.

I walk down the same street.
There is a deep hole in the sidewalk.
I walk around it.

I walk down another street."

From *There's a Hole in My Sidewalk: The Romance of Self-Discovery*

There are no shortcuts to becoming the person you're supposed to be, finding the right person to fuck included. The only way forward is to walk through the hellfire, get intimate with who you are, and risk taking responsibility for a part of you that can only be expressed sexually. Lose the Ambivalence keeping you from your Sexual Intuition, and you will get your life.

3.7: So You Got Laid, Now What?

When I first returned to dating post-wait-are-we-in-a-relationship-now-or-what-even-is-this-is-exactly-I know-we-hooked-up-once-but-then-I-didn't-hear-from-you-for-a-week-and-now-you're-texting-me-at-11 p.m.-on-a-Thursday... I've had to, to put it mildly, adjust. What I learned—and now coach people on—is that getting laid can be managed the same way people manage other things in their lives. If you have some fears about how you're going to handle yourself once you do get laid, this chapter is for you.

Many of us retreat into *avoidance* of sex or intimacy as a workaround for how scary it can be to get involved with someone. When you get burned, it's tough to get excited about putting your hand back on the hot sexy stove. Now is the time to develop some emotional oven mitts.

Let's talk about that fine quality designer drug readily available in your own brain called oxytocin. Oxytocin is called 'The Love Chemical,' partly because it's released on orgasm (as well as in some other situations, like breastfeeding, falling in love, and even *gloating*). Studies at the University of Haifa (using oxytocin nasal spray believe it or not) suggest this is one area where biological differences do play a part, but that doesn't mean these will necessarily predict someone's behavior. For some, oxytocin may inconveniently bond them with someone they're not necessarily going to see again, for others a competitive instinct can kick in that may still inspire wanting a rematch. Either way, it's potent and somewhat unpredictable.

If you find out (or know already) that you're the kind of person who gets a little 'carried away' with someone once they've made you 'oxytocin,' you can prepare for this eventuality by being more direct than your mother raised you to be (even though I'm sure your mother is a great lady. Ditto if your mother isn't a lady.)

A poly person once told me it takes 7 days to 'de-bond' from a person once you've slept with them. I haven't been able to find any data about this, but it always felt intuitively correct for me. If you know you get attached to someone quickly and your freshly sexed friend is not 'up for a relationship,' no matter how much you enjoyed yourself, *don't see them more often than every week, or even once every two weeks.*

This is an example of creating a 'structure' that works for you—based on how scorching hot, special, or promising the connection is—that minimizes any drama. After sex, you might already be planning a trip to every National Park on your tandem bicycle. You may be ready to feed each other fondue, to the exclusion of any fondue-related activities with others. You might just be gung-ho AF and that's great! But if you figure out that you/them/ both of you are not down for a longer-term journey, then don't buy a fondue set.

Put some effort into considering what *minimum* response is that you need to feel good, then communicate it *before* you sleep with them and *reiterate* it after the post-coital dust settles. This may be something as simple as needing a friendly text the next day or keeping things on the DL on social media. While I'm not into anything that even sounds like 'dating rules' or 'texting rules' or any of that horseshit, I am pro setting personal guidelines without being too freaked out if the other person can't follow them. Don't indulge in fantasies of the 'potential' of a relationship vs. the reality of what someone is offering. The trap to avoid is the uncovered manhole called, 'I can change someone.'

Generally I've found it's a good idea to develop iron self-discipline when it comes to texting. A rule I set for myself a long time ago, and recommend to clients, is never text anyone if you can't handle *any* outcome. Really play it out in your mind, them not texting back or responding with something less than ideal, and see if you would be *okay* or tearing your hair out. If it would be a hair-tearing scenario, take it as a sign that you're too attached to a result (or some Idea of that person) and **don't text**. Maybe you won't be as hooked tomorrow, but right now that's where it's at. (If someone does get nasty **do not engage**, you don't owe them anything.)

In my personal experience, and that of clients and friends over the years, I've found that if you're going to fuck again, it will happen. Sooner, later, or in a year when someone circles back around like a horny seagull (at which time you may already be doing it with another, sexier seagull). And they might just come knocking right at the moment it dawns on you that you won't be *dead* if they don't. This is my truth. Your intuition should guide you to *your* truth.

Also, I never text more than twice. I don't mind texting first, because I don't trip out about reaching out if I want to see them again. And then a follow up within an appropriate amount of time to make sure someone got my text. After that, if I know I don't have the stomach to handle silence, I don't give someone a chance to give me any. Your tolerance may be different and your results may vary, what matters is that you're setting up principles that make sense to you. This is not the same as some kind of manipulative 'rules,' it's knowing what makes you freak out and then ensuring that no matter how good it was to get laid, another person won't throw you off your game.

Even if you get ghosted, knowing you followed your personal protocol makes it sting less. Oh well. *Next...* There is an expression, "Rejection is God's Protection," and even if you're not religious, always, *always* consider someone who left your life as the Universe's way of protecting you from them. (If you believe that person was your 'Twin Flame,' soulmate, or last chance at happiness, that saying applies *double*.) I tell myself if I don't hear from someone that they definitely got hit by lightning and are in a coma, so sad. On the upside, we got laid!

Sometimes we put our lives on hold because we're waiting for a text or a message, or some other kind of validation that gives us permission to move forward. We pine and obsess and avoid our lives because what we had with that person is more exciting than laundry. We get tripped up trying to understand 'what happened' because the sex touched a nerve. This may even be why you stopped trying to get laid in the first place, because you decided you 'can't handle it.'

If you've been involved in sexual relationships with people who were Ambivalent, you may have experienced a "Come here, go away" phenomenon repeated in circles that drove one or both of you up a wall. Some call this 'love addiction,' aka a compulsion towards people we feel aren't good for us. Why couldn't you anticipate that person would string you along that way? How couldn't you see that this person was a predator/going to drive you bananas? WTF is wrong with this motherfucker anyway?

Did this cause you to lose faith in your own judgment? I'm here to give that faith back to you! You were doing the best you could with what you knew, and now the only thing left to do is forgive, both yourself and them (see:

burning effigies in well-ventilated areas.) From this point forward, resolve to be in touch with your own needs and personality enough to know what unequivocally won't work for you, and negotiate something better.

Maybe you think it's 'unromantic' or 'showing your hand' to have to negotiate when it comes to sex, but this ain't the 1950s and if you want to fuck like a grown-up, ya gotta act like one. This is an area where people involved in alternative lifestyles like polyamory and BDSM are a great example. We have to define and be specific about what we want because there *is* no set path, and obviously even more so if there's going to be some form of consensual pain involved. These black-belt communication skills are just as necessary in the 'vanilla' world, just not as valued, but getting laid makes them *worth it*.

Pre-sex I've had potential sexers intimate they were *totally* willing to take my kids to Little League (they weren't, and my intuition knew it, but it didn't matter because I didn't want them for that.) People can say all kinds of things to get laid, and that's fine, but what are the post-sex *facts*? How often do they call/text? Do they show up when and where they say they will?

How does your body feel in their presence? Do they make you feel tired?

I don't advocate setting up a 'structure' with someone if their texts make your stomach hurt, or if you're being coerced, manipulated, or abused. Ditto if someone bores you deeply for reasons you can't fathom. You can allow for the possibility of sex becoming more passionate the *more* you know someone, but only if it's all happening in a way (and at a pace) that works for you. The somatic intelligence you started working on earlier in this book will help you ascertain if that stomach sensation is a benign love-ache, or your gut telling you to get the fuck out.

If you sleep with someone and despite what you anticipated (or confirming what you kinda already knew) you're really *not* into it, be as kind and honest as possible. Either way, you don't have feel desperate, even if your radar was a bit off on this occasion, you can trust that what you learned will guide you to someone who is a better fit.

One other way to get real is when it comes to alcohol. In a fair and just world, we would all be able to get loaded and go where we want, to fuck whomever we please. Unfortunately, for many people, this is not reality. Know what alcohol does to your power of choice, and act accordingly. Remember, if you have to 'loosen up' anything to the extent that you don't have full control over your decisions, this is not a sustainable approach.

So there it is, the guide for getting laid like a badass that was inside you all along, Dorothy. You've stopped branding your sexual urges as negative, done some work identifying your Needs, and are ready to take actions IRL and/or online. You're questioning your old Torture Loops and Ideas, reveling in your Fuck Energy, and sensing others' beyond just the Cerebral, Emotional or Genital. You've set your Fuck Frequency, are feeling yourself (in *every* way) and have entered the Fuck Zone. You're dealing with your Fuck Trauma because fuck trauma, seriously. You know what you're available for, and you're aware of where Ambivalence might stop you. Powered by Sexual Intuition, reality is not something that needs to be avoided, just the canvas on which to manifest our colorful, Fuck Motivated selves. And what could be hotter than that?

Glossary and Context of Terms

AF: As fuck (i.e. very much so.)

Aftercare: The pampering or comforting attention given to a partner (usually the submissive) at the end of a 'scene' or experience in BDSM.

Ambivalence: A state of being that stays conflicted about dating and relationship choices.

Asexual: Someone who doesn't experience sexual attraction.

Attachment: The Buddhist reminder that it is damaging to hold too tightly to a person, place, or possession, and not to value the result over the journey.

BDSM: Bondage/Discipline, Dominance/submission, Sadism/Masochism

Cerebral (n.): Someone who picks whose relationship choices are intellectual, based solely on rational criteria.

Cis/cisgender: people who identify with the sex they were assigned at birth.

Conscious: Approaching life in an intentional way, as opposed to literally 'not in a coma.'

Demisexual: Someone who doesn't often experience sexual attraction without an emotional bond, but not asexual (see: not Fuck Motivated.)

DBT: Dialectical behavioral therapy, a modality developed by Marsha Linehan to help people with trauma and other mental/emotional glitches.

Deviant: Someone whose sexual practices vary from the 'norm,' whatever that is. (I don't use this in a negative context if the deviance is consensual.)

Emotional (n.): Someone who picks potential partners using completely heart-centered criteria.

Energy: The particular vibe a person emits or their essence, discovered by Fritz Albert-Popp PhD, and measurable by such controversial means as Kirlian photography.

Fetish: An intense sexual arousal towards a very specific practice or thing. (Also known as paraphilia.)

Fetlife: Fetlife.com is considered the kinky Facebook, though people's 'friend requests' tend to be far more explicit. Check it out if you're not easily offended.

Fuck Energy: The movement of desire in the body, which radiates to others.

Fuck Frequency: The impression of your and other people's sexuality, based on what you broadcast to the world with your words, Fuck Energy, and behavior.

Fuck Motivated: The degree to which your actions and choices are motived by sex at the present time.

Fuck Zone: A way of seeing the world where everything and everyone is sexy.

Genital (n.): Someone who picks whom to date, have sex with, or marry using a physical or genital-centered criteria.

Idea: A rigid impression formed in early or later life that limits a person from achieving freedom of choice, especially in sex and dating.

IED: Improvised explosive device, an unconventional bomb often used on roadsides that are designed to be difficult to spot and cause maximum harm.

IRL: In real life.

Kundalini awakening: Awakening a dormant form of primal energy through breathing, meditation, yoga, or Tantra practices.

217

Limerance: The exciting, hormone-fuelled excitement at the beginning of a relationship.

LTR: Long term relationship.

Marrieds: Married people.

Monagamish: A relationship model coined by Dan Savage that is not completely monogamous, but still with a primary partner.

NBD: No big deal.

Needs: The driving essentials you can't do without, especially in relationships.

Newb: Newbie, someone without a lot of sexual experience.

Obvi: Obviously.

On the regular: Regularly.

Pervert/perv: Someone in to 'unusual' sexual practices (again, without the dictionary's negative connotation.)

Psychic Shrapnel: Disturbing thought fragments left over from another time and place.

Queer: A gender-inclusive umbrella term for people who are not heterosexual.

RN: Right now.

Sexual Intuition: A sixth sense about what you need sexually, and the ability to attract others with dovetailing needs.

SOL: Shit out of luck.

Somatic Experience Processing: A modality of therapy that focuses on sensations in the body.

STIs: Sexually transmitted infections: At the time of this writing, the terminology is moving away from the term 'sexually transmitted diseases' because of the negative connotations of the word 'disease.' Technically you're 'infected' with STDs, and can infect others, so they all qualify as STIs.

Torture Loops: The endless cycle of obsessive, negative thoughts.

Trampage: Rampage of being a 'tramp.' (See: Fuck Motivated.)

Vanilla: Not kinky, 'conventional' sexual practices.

Youngs: Young people.

Acknowledgements

Thank you from my heart to sex ed superstar Sunny Megatron, who provided genius feedback, as well as much-needed laughs in between making sure I drilled down into what I was getting at with sensitivity. Thanks also to my first editor Isabelle Kohn, a gifted sex writer with a grammar fetish.

My clients are my greatest spiritual teachers. Thank you for entrusting me with holding space for you—I'm honored and grateful. Thanks to all the people who were welcoming, helpful, and encouraging in the sex ed world: Tristan Taormino, Elle Chase, Hudsy Hawn, Hercules Liotard, Wry Mantione, Buck Angel, Mickey Mod, Jess Nalu, Ashley Manta, everyone at SHELA, and Emily Morse.

I'm grateful for faith in my writing and coaching endeavors from Lisa Short, Rose Greenberg, Brett Parker, Angela Berliner, Kathryn Alice, Toni Torres, Marnie Sehayek, Melissa Broder, Lori Dome, Dana Johnson, Amy Dresner, Alina Sack, John Fugelsang, and every reader who has ever responded positively to my writing, thank you, it mattered!

And posthumous thanks to Psalm Isadora, who inspired me in ways I cannot fathom.

70227737R00124

Made in the USA
San Bernardino, CA
26 February 2018